THE COMPLETE
PLAB

Objective
Structured
Clinical
Examination

Commissioning Editor: Laurence Hunter
Project Development Manager: Siân Jarman
Project Manager: Nancy Arnott
Designer: Sarah Russell

THE COMPLETE
PLAB

Objective Structured Clinical Examination

Dr M Afzal Mir
Senior Lecturer & Consultant Physician
Department of Medicine
University of Wales College of Medicine
Cardiff

Dr Srinivasan Madhusudan
Specialist Registrar in Medical Oncology
Oxford Radcliffe Hospitals NHS Trust
Oxford

Dr E Anne Freeman
Consultant Physician
Care of the Elderly Department
St Woolos and Royal Gwent Hospitals
Newport, Gwent

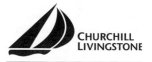

CHURCHILL
LIVINGSTONE

EDINBURGH LONDON NEW YORK PHILADELPHIA ST LOUIS SYDNEY TORONTO 2003

CHURCHILL LIVINGSTONE
An imprint of Elsevier Science Limited

First published 2003

ISBN 0-443-07050-4

British Library Cataloguing in Publication Data
A catalogue record for this book is available from the British Library.

Library of Congress Cataloging in Publication Data
A catalog record for this book is available from the Library of Congress.

Note
Medical knowledge is constantly changing. As new information becomes available,
changes in treatment, procedures, equipment and the use of drugs become
necessary. The authors and the publishers have taken care to ensure that the
information given in this text is accurate and up to date. However, readers are
strongly advised to confirm that the information, especially with regard to drug
usage, complies with the latest legislation and standards of practice.

ELSEVIER
SCIENCE

your source for books,
journals and multimedia
in the health sciences

www.elsevierhealth.com

The
publisher's
policy is to use
**paper manufactured
from sustainable forests**

Printed in China by RDC Group Limited

Preface

The practical, or Part 2, test for the Professional and Linguistics Assessments Board (PLAB) examination is a critical assessment of bedside behaviour and clinical examination technique. Although it has no formal syllabus, its content and requirements are well known and transparent. The failure rate remains high even though the tasks set in this exam are the ones that all candidates are expected to have learned during their undergraduate years. The reason for these poor results is that in this exam candidates face several hurdles, testing not only their medical knowledge, but communication skills, bedside behaviour, professionalism, and practical techniques.

Candidates may be asked to take a history, provide counselling to a patient with a particular illness or disability, examine a system or subsystem, and carry out procedures under the watchful eyes of the examiners. Although these tasks can be performed easily in the privacy of a side room on a one-to-one basis, the presence of the examiners and the exam setting itself can prove unnerving even for well-prepared candidates. The use of a manikin instead of a responsive, and often sympathetic, human subject presents an additional problem to many candidates who cannot relate to an inanimate object. While it is true that these skills can only be acquired by constant practice with patients, friends and manikins, there has been a need for a book which provides step-by-step guidance in the various aspects of the wide spectrum of tasks that all postgraduate doctors are expected to perform. We have endeavoured to accomplish this objective by basing this book on our own experience, and on information collected from candidates, examiners and tutors for this exam.

In Section 1 we have given some general advice on how to prepare for this exam, and on the format of the objective structured clinical examination (OSCE), with samples of the clinical scenarios and procedures which are often asked about. Section 2 contains a collection of histories that cover most of the likely scenarios in the exam. For each scenario we have suggested a differential diagnosis, outlined a problem-solving approach, and provided a list of questions which would narrow down the possibilities. In Section 3 there is a selection of counselling scenarios and information on pamphlets and counselling agencies available in the UK. Section 4 presents 25 examination techniques and Section 5 covers 26 procedures. Sections 4 and 5 are supported by numerous illustrations, which should ease the learning process.

Although this book has been directed at the PLAB examination, its teaching on communication skills, problem-solving history taking, counselling, examination techniques, and on procedures is also relevant to medical students and junior doctors (internees) in their everyday practice and should prove to be a useful aid on the wards.

Cardiff   M.A.M.

2003   E.A.F.

                                                                 S.M.

Acknowledgements

The pictures demonstrating clinical skills and procedures were specially produced in the Media Resource Centre and Clinical Skills Laboratory, University Hospital of Wales, Cardiff. We are indebted to Messrs Keith Bellamy and Paul Crompton and Ms Bolette Jones, whose skills and perseverance were responsible for the fine quality of pictures used in this book. Our thanks are due to Professor Richard Morton and Mr Keith Richardson for allowing us the use of the Resource Centre and the Clinical Skills Laboratory.

We are grateful to all those listed below who read the individual scenarios and generously gave us their useful advice: Mr Nazar Amso, Dr Mani Baines, Dr Sam Bando, Dr Jacob Easaw, Dr Mark Evans, Dr Peter Holt, Dr Tom Hughes, Dr Dean Jenkins, Dr Pushpa Jinadev, Dr Ayub Mirza, Dr Manzoor Malik, Dr Jamuna Mysore, Mr Sibaprasad Senapati and Mr David Teanan.

Contents

Preparation for the Objective Structured Clinical Examination (OSCE)

The Part 2 PLAB examination

The Part 2 PLAB exam is a comprehensive test of a medical graduate's competence in: obtaining a problem-solving history; performing a slick and purposeful examination; counselling patients about their illness and before discharging them from hospital; and performing everyday practical procedures. A competent performance in this exam requires knowledge of how to obtain succinct histories, the acquisition of clinical skills, experience in counselling patients, practical experience in carrying out procedures, and a good command of the English language. For any hope of a successful outcome in this exam, candidates need thorough preparation by polishing up their skills.

Preparation

Doctors approaching this exam would be expected to have already learned the basic clinical skills and procedures as undergraduates and in their early postgraduate years. However, many of them may not have achieved spontaneity in performing these skills; some may be deficient in performing some of the required procedures; and many may be unsure of their communication skills. We would suggest that this book should be used for brushing up on all the skills you have learned and for filling in the gaps in your repertoire.

Learn during attachments

Medical students overseas who are contemplating taking the PLAB exam after their graduation should see as many patients as they can during their clinical attachments and practise history-taking and examination routines. Whenever possible, go on consultant ward rounds and observe how they discuss their patients' illnesses, management and prognosis with them. Read the relevant sections on history-taking and on counselling in this book as you encounter them on the wards and practise these on patients, friends, toy dolls and in front of a mirror.

Doctors who obtain clinical attachments in the UK before the exam should not only brush up on their clinical skills, but should also be on the lookout for any opportunity for eavesdropping on communication sessions between senior doctors and their patients. This can easily be arranged with the doctors concerned when they are planning to have a chat with their patients in the privacy of a side room. Permission must be sought from the patients before you decide to sit in with them. Read the counselling section in this book and explore what patient information material the hospital provides, familiarizing yourself with what counselling resources and aids are available. Practise counselling skills with your colleagues on a one-to-one basis.

Do not miss learning opportunities, such as clinical meetings and grand rounds, as these will help you to increase your knowledge and improve your presentation. Make sure that you observe any procedures (e.g. lumbar puncture, chest drainage, ascitic tap, arterial blood gases, etc.) that are being undertaken in your hospital.

Practise clinical skills

Clinical skills such as palpation, percussion and eliciting reflexes look deceptively easy when an expert is at work but, in reality, it takes many years of practice to achieve such a level of competence. Even at the higher medical exams it is not uncommon to see a doctor using a tendon hammer as if swatting flies, or using the force of the whole forearm in percussion. Inadequate and clumsy methods look unseemly and create an unfavourable impression on the examiners.

Do not take for granted that your clinical skills are either already adequate or that you will acquire the necessary finesse with experience. Incorrect methods remain incorrect even though they may look less clumsy with experience. Learn the correct methods from your tutors and senior doctors at the outset and practise them on your colleagues or toy dolls. There are videotapes on basic clinical skills in the libraries of most hospitals in this country: study these and then practise them repeatedly until you acquire a smooth technique.

Learn examination sequences

The examiners expect you to carry out a step-by-step examination in the conventional order when they ask you to examine a system. It looks bad if you jump back and forth from one step to another in a haphazard manner, or appear to be undecided about what to do next. Examiners have been known to ask students, for example, whether the pulse was of a collapsing character at the end of their presentation, knowing that the candidates had failed to check for it. You should adhere to the conventional examination routines and practise them until they become second nature. Thus, if you are woken up during the night and asked to examine the neurological integrity of a patient's legs, you should be able to follow the sequence unhesitatingly — bulk, tone, power, coordination, abnormal movements, reflexes, sensations, and gait. For a step-by-step guide to examination routines, you may also consider consulting Mir: *Atlas of Clinical Skills*, Saunders, London, 1997.

Using this book

This book contains a wide variety of material covering all aspects of the Part 2 PLAB exam. The four principal sections cover most of the common clinical scenarios, problems, examination routines, and procedures that we meet in everyday clinical practice and the ones that are commonly encountered in the exam.

Histories

We have provided a comprehensive selection of histories, with differential diagnoses and the questions you may ask, covering common complaints in medicine, surgery, gynaecology and obstetrics, paediatrics, and psychiatry. Go over these carefully and work out your line of questioning for each symptom. Consider supplementary questions which might follow on from any of the different answers the patient might give you. Doctors from the Indian subcontinent and the Middle East are at a disadvantage in history-taking because patients from these countries expect their doctors to diagnose their illnesses without asking too many questions. In contrast, Western patients welcome detailed enquiry and usually give answers as outlined in a standard textbook!

Practise your questioning routine for common complaints with a colleague, preferably someone who is preparing for the same exam. After you have taken a history, practise summarizing your conclusions and presenting these to the examiner in an articulate and confident manner.

Examination routines

In Section 4 we have described the clinical examination routines (each in conventional order), supported by clinical photographs and illustrations, for all systems and major subsystems. You can adapt these to your individual methods and style but do ensure that you do not omit an important step. Practise them on patients and colleagues as often as possible, or even on toy dolls or pillows if a volunteer is not readily available.

Practising on dolls can be quite useful as the examiners often use manikins in this exam. Unless you are familiar with treating the manikins as real patients you may be flummoxed when asked to talk to or examine one. Remember, the examiners are

treating them as real patients when they introduce them to you
— *This is Mr Smith. Please examine his chest.* Your approach is all-
important: you should introduce yourself to him, ask for his
permission to examine him, and engage him in a brief, pleasant
conversation, as suggested in the cases described. Always bear in
mind that you are examining a real patient. Now and again, tell
him what you are doing, or are about to do, and ask for his
permission for any special manoeuvres such as when you adjust
his backrest when examining his heart, or when you are
reaching down to the groin to feel for the femoral pulse or for
an inguinal hernia. Learn to be as gentle with the manikin as
you would be with a real patient — treat it with respect, partially
cover it with the sheet when you have finished examining it, and
thank it as if it is a real patient.

In short, practise all the examination routines given in this
book on patients or inanimate objects with delicacy and care. You
should practise them repeatedly until you become step-perfect so
that you can reproduce them in the correct sequence with
spontaneity and fluency. A useful way of imprinting the routines
on your memory is to repeat the *whole* sequence every time you
miss a step, and keep doing this until you miss nothing.

Procedures

We have given detailed descriptions of 26 procedures which we
believe a junior doctor should be proficient in. In addition to
the ones that are usually asked for in the exam (e.g. peripheral
vein cannulation, suturing, catheterization, etc.), we have
included some others (e.g. insertion of a chest drain, fine-needle
aspiration) because you will need to know these as a junior
doctor. For each procedure we have explained its purpose,
suggested how you will need to explain it to the patient, and
provided a step-by-step practical description of the technique.
We suggest that you practise all these procedures on a manikin,
including the ones you have done before. In most teaching
hospitals in this country there are Clinical Skills Laboratories,
and if you approach a friendly tutor there you may get to
practise some of these procedures on a suitable manikin. We
have illustrated some of the procedures, particularly when we
felt that the text needed some support (e.g. tying a knot), and
we would suggest that you practise the steps that you are not
fully familiar with.

Counselling

This is by far the most difficult part of the exam, mainly because sensitive and effective communication is a skill that takes some considerable time to acquire. Even expert clinicians find that giving bad news or exploring a sensitive area never becomes any easier with experience. In this country communication skills have only recently been incorporated into the curriculum; most PLAB candidates come from Eastern countries where the old perception of 'the doctor knows best' still prevails.

Obviously, communication skills cannot be acquired in a short preparatory period before the exam but you can make substantial progress by rehearsing some of the common situations described in Section 3. You need to have a reasonable command of English but remember that even a limited vocabulary can be put to good use if you speak slowly and clearly and use simple terms. You also need an adequate knowledge of each condition. With these considerations in mind, study each scenario, get hold of any pamphlets and patient information sheets about the condition from a local hospital, speak to the relevant specialist nurses and counsellors, and practise delivering a short spiel first to yourself and then to a colleague.

There are some general points that are worth taking on board. Find out what, or how much, the patient knows and build on that. Encourage him to ask questions. Deliver bad news with compassion and sensitivity. You may use a gentle opening statement such as, 'I'm afraid I have some bad news', or 'I'm afraid there is no easy way of saying this.' A simple rule of thumb is that each piece of bad news must be accompanied by a 'but'. For example, if you tell the patient that he has a lymphoma, you might add, '*but* there are some effective treatments available'. We have given some more useful suggestions at the beginning of Section 3. Suffice it to say here that you should prepare a short spiel for each common clinical scenario and practise delivering it.

Psychological preparation

Part 2 of the PLAB exam is a confrontational exercise in which a candidate has to perform in front of the watchful eyes of the examiners. Our enquiries have revealed that many candidates lack confidence and that even the knowledgeable ones appear hesitant in their interchanges with the examiners. Their anxiety to do better only compounds their nervousness and they find themselves on a downward slope, losing their self-belief and so their composure, which undermines their performance. This may be partly because in their country of origin the senior academic staff are regarded (also by themselves) as tin gods, keeping their distance from the junior staff and students who rarely speak unless spoken to. This restraint becomes a major handicap when such candidates encounter unfamiliar senior academics as examiners.

The other problem is that Indian and Middle-Eastern English differs in idiom and expression from the language spoken here, and most overseas graduates think in their own language and then translate it into English when speaking to an examiner or a patient. For example, 'please' and 'thank you' are incorporated into sentences in most Indian languages and are not spoken as additional words as in Western languages. Even the most polite Indian doctor may sound rude if he thinks in Hindi and speaks in English! This problem, together with differences in kinetic behaviour often results in a disharmonious exchange in the exam.

To develop a good psychological approach to this exam, take these considerations into account and, after full preparation as suggested above, go into the exam with the intention of speaking confidently and clearly as you would to a senior colleague. The examiners are there to test your clinical competence as prescribed by the General Medical Council, and as detailed in this book; they do not expect obsequious behaviour.

Remember that you do not get a mark for what you know unless you say it to the examiners and you do the tasks asked of you. The examiners have a pre-printed mark sheet for each task and they have to tick each component of the task as you perform it. For example, if your task is to take a history from a patient with a headache, there will be marks on the sheet not only for how comprehensively you cover headache but also for how you develop a rapport with the patient and how you treat him. Study the General Medical Council's booklet, *The PLAB Test, Part 2, Advice to Candidates*, which explains the structure of the exam and gives useful advice.

If you prepare along the lines suggested, study this book thoroughly, and practise the examination routines and procedures, then there is no reason why you cannot give a good account of yourself. Remind yourself of that before you go into the exam.

The Objective Structured Clinical Examination (OSCE)

The OSCE format is designed to make the assessment both objective and fair. At each station there is the same patient, volunteer, or manikin; the same examiner (sometimes accompanied by an observer); the same time allowed (currently 5 minutes); and the same set of marking criteria. Examiners are directed to apply these criteria without allowing themselves to be influenced by their subjective impressions. At each station you will be expected to complete a task (history-taking, counselling, examination or a procedure) watched by an examiner who will not interfere or comment, but who at the end will listen to your conclusions, possibly ask a question or two, before ticking the pre-printed mark sheet.

Here we describe a typical 16-station format which is used at all centres. Every candidate will be expected to carry out cardiopulmonary resuscitation at one of these stations to the examiners' satisfaction. Mercifully, two of these stations are for rest where you have some time for restoration and reflection. One of the two rest stations may be a pilot station where you will be given a task to do but it will be a practice slot and you will not be marked for it. The rest stations are clearly marked.

Station I

Talk to Mr Hopkirk who is about to be discharged from hospital after an acute myocardial infarction.

You may be given a pamphlet and asked to go through it with the patient. Examiners will often point out one or two issues that are not mentioned in the pamphlet and ask you to discuss these with the patient and give him appropriate advice. This applies particularly to drugs prescribed for the patient which may not be detailed in the pamphlet and you will be expected to advise him as you would when discharging one of your own patients. Do not forget to greet the patient and introduce yourself, and to thank him before you leave the cubicle.

Station II

Examine the fundus of this patient.

There is usually a manikin at this station. You may choose to address your greeting, introductory comments and explanations to the examiner, but you should not omit these to the manikin. As you proceed to fundoscopy they will project one of the commonly seen retinopathies, for example those associated with diabetes mellitus or hypertension. The examiner will ask you to describe the findings and to give the diagnosis.

Station III

You are told that you are an SHO in paediatrics or casualty and you are being telephoned by an anxious mother whose child has a fever and a rash.

The unexpected structure of this scenario unsettles many candidates, but the well-prepared candidate will be equal to the task. Reassure the mother, saying that you will do everything you can to help. Take a brief history from her, asking, for example, about the onset of the fever and rash; any other symptoms such as vomiting or headache; the condition of the child; and a description of the rash. Some candidates have even asked the mother to do the 'tumbler test' on the rash to see if it fades when a glass is pressed on it.

At the end you may have to settle on the diagnosis of meningococcaemia. Explain to the mother that the child may have 'brain fever' but that this is eminently treatable, and that she should get him to the hospital as soon as possible.

Station IV

Collect blood samples from this patient for a full blood count, urea and electrolytes, and plasma glucose. Please label the containers and fill in the relevant laboratory forms.

This 'patient' is invariably a manikin primed with blood. The process is fairly straightforward (see p. 383). You will be expected to explain the procedure to the manikin, collect the blood samples and put them in the correct containers, remembering that the sample for plasma glucose has to go in a special container. The patient details must be correctly written on the containers as well as on the request forms. Be careful to discard the needles in the sharps bin.

Station V

This is a rest station where you can relax until the next bell.

Station VI

Collect a cervical smear from this patient.

This instruction is deceptively simple as the procedure of using a speculum, obtaining a smear from the correct area and the preparation of slides (see p. 438) requires a considerable degree of experience. The patient is a manikin at every centre and the examiner will be watching every step without giving you any feedback.

Station VII

Perform cardiopulmonary resuscitation on this patient who has just collapsed.

This is an important station as the candidates who fail to satisfy the examiners here will fail the whole exam, irrespective of their performance at other stations. The examiners will observe silently without any comments. Make sure that you have learned to perform all the steps in sequence (see p. 372) before you go to the exam — the omission of any step (e.g. exposing the chest of the manikin before starting cardiac massage) will result in failure.

Station VIII

This is Mr Hudson, who has been complaining of giddiness. Please measure his blood pressure.

There is always a volunteer at this station, which makes it easy to greet him, to introduce yourself and to explain the procedure. These pleasantries will enable you to keep the patient resting in a chair for at least 2 minutes before you measure his blood pressure — it is worth making a point of this by asking the patient if he has been resting for a few minutes before you entered the cubicle. There are two further considerations worthy of note. First, you will be provided with a stethoscope with four earpieces and the examiner will be listening simultaneously with you for the Korotkoff sounds. This need not disturb you but you will have to make sure that you identify correctly phases 1, 4 and 5. Second, although it should be self-evident here that in a patient with giddiness you should look for postural hypotension, it is advisable to measure both the sitting and standing blood pressures irrespective of the presenting complaint.

Station IX

Examine this patient's second to seventh cranial nerves and explain each step to me as you go through the examination.

In most cases there will be a volunteer at this station with no cranial nerve deficit. The purpose of the exercise is to see if you are able to explain the process both to the patient and to the examiner and can perform the necessary steps of the examination (see p. 287). A useful way of doing this would be to explain each main step to the examiner and then explain the mechanics of your tests to the patient. For example, you would say to the examiner that you wish to examine the second cranial nerve which involves testing visual acuity, central, peripheral, and colour vision, and the afferent limb of the pupillary light reflex, and then explain each step to the patient as you proceed with your examination.

Station X

This is a rest station where you can relax until the next bell.

Station XI

This is Mrs Pemberton, who has had palpitations. Take a history from her.

This is the first of the three history stations. You will need to explore the main complaint; any associated symptoms; and important aspects of the past medical, family, and social history. Your presentation should include a tentative diagnosis for the palpitations (e.g. sinus tachycardia, ectopics, atrial fibrillation, supraventricular tachycardia); suggestions about underlying reasons (anxiety state, any cardiac lesion, etc.); which (reasonable) investigations you might arrange (e.g. ECG, ambulatory ECG monitoring); and some comments on possible management strategies.

Station XII

Take a history from this 26-year-old man who presented with left-sided chest pain and give a differential diagnosis.

There may be a volunteer at this station who has been given an information sheet which he will have studied, enabling him to answer your questions. After exploring the characteristics of the pain (site, nature, radiation, relation to respiration, aggravating and relieving factors) and any associated symptoms, you will need to cover other aspects of past medical, family, social, and drug history. The differential diagnosis will include musculoskeletal pain, pleurisy, spontaneous pneumothorax, herpes zoster, pulmonary infarction, and pneumonia, depending on the answers given by the patient.

Station XIII

Mr Ambridge has been referred to your Rheumatology Clinic with a pain in his left big toe. Take a short history and give a differential diagnosis.

With gout, osteoarthrosis, injury, and infection at the top of your list, you will need to obtain a full history of the pain and ask if he has any swelling, fever, or involvement of other joints, and if he has been given any drugs (e.g. diuretics) recently. Even though you have been asked to take a short history there should be enough time to ask the patient whether he has had any similar episodes in the past and whether there is any family history of gout.

Station XIV

Mr Turner is complaining of cough and breathlessness. Please examine his chest.

This sounds reasonably straightforward but remember that you have to develop a good rapport with the patient as well as demonstrate your competence in all four components of a standard examination (inspection, palpation, percussion and auscultation) in only 5 minutes. If you have practised your examination routines, you should not have any major problems.

Station XV

Mr Smith has sustained a cut on his arm. Please suture it.

At this station, there will be a manikin arm with a clean cut with two flaps ready to be sutured. You may even notice previous needle marks and the impressions made by the silk thread. Although a manikin arm is easily accessible and will not withdraw with pain, suturing its plastic flaps can prove tricky.

Hold the needle with the needle holder closer to its sharp end in order to get better control as you pierce the flap. It is worth practising this on a minikin before you go to the examination.

Station XVI

Get a consent form signed by Mrs Armitage for an autopsy on her father who died recently in hospital of an unknown cause.

This can prove to be an awkward task and you will need all the patience that you can muster. Mrs Armitage will be an actress (who may be prone to fits of overacting!). She may be visibly upset and you must forget that she is an actress and start playing *your* part, consoling her as sympathetically as possible. Do not mention the autopsy until you have restored her to some degree of equilibrium. Tell her that you are sorry that despite modern advances in medicine you and your colleagues were unable to save her father's life. Tell her that her father's illness was severe and his deterioration rapid, or that his constitution was too weak, or that because you did not know the cause of his illness, it was not possible to provide the appropriate treatment in time. This last suggestion would provide you with an opportunity to ask for her permission for an autopsy.

Do not be in a hurry to demand a signature: the purpose of the exercise is to see how you will handle this situation. You will have plenty of time so use it wisely to console her and to explain the need for an autopsy. Explain that you need to know why he died. Explain that this will not bring him back but that the knowledge gained may prevent someone else's death, that it would be a service to medicine and mankind. Be sure to add that she should not feel under any obligation, legal or moral, but that an autopsy would reveal the cause of her father's death. She may use emotive language and claim that you are going to disfigure her father, carve him up or saw his head. You must admit that some cutting is necessary to examine the internal organs but that it is done without compromising human dignity, and that all cuts are neatly sutured to restore the body to its original form.

History taking

Introduction

History-taking is a fundamental aspect of clinical work and all subsequent patient experiences, either in hospital or at home, are based on the very first interview with a doctor. The aim of this first interchange is to obtain an accurate account of the symptoms, which may provide clues about the underlying clinical problem and insight into how it is affecting the patient. History-taking is an art and all good clinicians constantly strive to improve this skill throughout their clinical career. Even recent medical graduates, however, while not yet having developed the niceties of the art, should have grasped the basic principles of a medical interview. They should be able to get an accurate account of a patient's complaints and be able to use this to reach a diagnosis.

The purpose of history-taking OSCE stations in the PLAB exam is to assess whether candidates, wishing to practise as internees in the UK, can take an effective history from the patient and make a competent initial clinical assessment. You enter the station when the bell rings where you will find a simulated or a real patient with the examiner. The patient will have been given a sheet clearly outlining what symptoms he is supposed to have and what answers he can give you. The examiner has a pre-printed checklist listing the principal components of history-taking (e.g. initial pleasantries and rapport; presenting complaints with their onset, progress, and response to any treatment; other history including past medical and family history, social and other relevant history; and diagnosis). The examiner will not interfere with your interviewing process but will observe whether or not you cover all the important aspects. When the 30-second bell rings he will ask you for a diagnosis.

Most postgraduate doctors know the fundamentals of history-taking and believe that they can cope with these encounters. However, the exam setting, the time limit, and the presence of the examiner (possibly with an observer) all add to the stress of having to take a history. Knowledge of what you are likely to encounter and some practice, however, will make you confident in your ability to obtain all the relevant facets of a history and draw the appropriate conclusions.

To help prepare you for this aspect of the exam we have presented 38 histories in this section, covering the most commonly encountered problems in clinical practice. Each case begins with the examiner's question. This is followed by a differential diagnosis which should enable you to sharpen your focus on the likely clinical problems and think of appropriate questions. Although these are described in the subsequent 'History' and 'Questions' sections, it would be more profitable for you to devise your own differential diagnosis and questioning strategies *before* you read any further than the examiner's opening statement. This exercise would sharpen your ability to respond quickly and logically to a set of complaints with a differential diagnosis and appropriate questions.

We have provided a suggested list of questions for each case both here and elsewhere in this book. This will be especially useful for candidates who experience difficulty in phrasing their questions in English. We have attempted to cover as many of the questions that may be required as possible. However, you will not need *all* the questions given in each case: after the first few questions, your subsequent enquiries will depend on what answers the 'patient' gives you.

After the initial pleasantries it is always a good strategy to ask the patient in a general way what his or her complaints are. Remember, these patients are not tutored to confuse or mislead you unless you yourself go off at a tangent into an area unfamiliar to them. This book should help you to concentrate your mind on the relevant differential diagnosis for each common complaint so that you do not ask the patient too many irrelevant questions and force him to abandon his script. Allowing the patient to phrase his complaints in his own words at the outset will give you some idea about the scope of your differential diagnosis and the other aspects of the history that you will need to cover. We suggest that you practise some of these scenarios with a colleague, alternately taking the roles of the patient and the candidate: this will help you to negotiate these stations with greater confidence.

Anne, a 17-year-old schoolgirl, has been brought to the doctor by her mother because she has had no periods. The mother is very worried that her daughter may have some 'gland trouble'. Please take a history.

Amenorrhoea is the absence of periods and can be classified as *primary* (not yet had the menarche) or *secondary* (cessation of periods some time after a normal menarche). As amenorrhoea is the only abnormality given, you should recall some of the principal causes and take the history in stages to focus on the probable underlying cause.

Common causes of amenorrhoea

Remember that the patient may be a late starter, a fitness fanatic, or may have a hormonal imbalance or an eating disorder.

Other major causes of amenorrhoea

Primary amenorrhoea

- Structural — imperforate hymen, congenital defects of uterus and vagina
- Ovarian failure — hypoplasia, chromosomal (Turner's syndrome)
- Hypothalamic–pituitary causes — tumours (craniopharyngioma, prolactinoma), infection, granuloma
- Endocrine and metabolic causes — Cushing's syndrome, Addison's disease, anorexia nervosa, malabsorption
- Chronic diseases — diabetes mellitus, tuberculosis

Secondary amenorrhoea
- Pregnancy
- Hypothalamic–pituitary — tumours, infection, granuloma, functional (depression, anorexia nervosa), post-pubertal hypothalamic hypogonadism
- Endocrine and metabolic — Cushing's syndrome, Addison's disease, thyroid disease, obesity, undernutrition (anorexia), malabsorption
- Chronic diseases — tuberculosis, connective tissue diseases

Skillful questioning should probe for any evidence of psychological disturbance and she should be asked about her dietary and exercise habits, lifestyle, personal and social stresses, any family history of genetic anomalies, and about her physical growth and development.

History

The story given suggests that this girl has primary amenorrhoea. The candidate should confirm this at the outset because the causes are slightly different from those for secondary amenorrhoea. Once you confirm that she has primary amenorrhoea you must still exclude *pregnancy*, which is the most common and important cause of secondary amenorrhoea. Although it is likely that the mother would have asked her daughter if she was pregnant before taking her to a doctor, you cannot assume this and in some cases one may have to ask the question directly.

If there is any suspicion that she has had a period in the past and that pregnancy may be the cause of her amenorrhoea she should be asked privately and with some sensitivity. After having established that this is primary amenorrhoea, the next thing to decide is if she is a 'late developer' with delayed puberty. The mother may have had delayed puberty as well so questions should be asked of them both. You then need to look for any other possible cause. Skillful questioning should probe into any evidence of psychological disturbance and she should be asked about her dietary and exercise habits and about her physical growth and development.

Gonadal dysgenesis is a possibility and abnormal/absent secondary sexual characteristics may give clues to an underlying cause, for example, Turner's syndrome, a chromosomal disorder (XO) with short stature (less than 5 feet), webbed neck,

Reader registration card

Please help us to improve the quality of our books by completing the following details and returning the card to us.

Book title and author/editor: _____

Your name: _____   Address: _____

Course name: _____   _____

Year of study: _____   _____

Position: _____   E-mail: _____

How did you hear about this book? (please tick appropriate box(es)):

☐ Direct mail from publisher ☐ Conference ☐ Book review ☐ Library ☐ Book

☐ Lecturer recommendation ☐ Peer recommendation ☐ Other (please specify)_____

Type of purchase: ☐ Individual ☐ Department ☐ Library ☐ Main library

Do you have any brief comments on this book? _____

For more information on titles or
to register to receive regular e-mail
updates on new titles please visit:

www.elsevierhealth.com

Please return this card to the address overleaf
No stamp required *if posted in the UK*
Or fax (outside the UK) to: + 44 20 8309 0807

ELSEVIER
SCIENCE

micrognathia, low-set ears, absent breasts, increased carrying angles, and paucity of axillary and pubic hair.

If the patient looks underweight and undernourished and there is a suspicion that she may have *anorexia nervosa* (a condition affecting girls and young women, who become obsessed with their body image and with losing weight) then you should consider asking the five questions from the SCOFF questionnaire (*see below*), in which one point is counted for every 'yes', and a score of two or more indicates a diagnosis of anorexia nervosa.

Questions

Are you sure you have never had any periods at all — not even a show on your underwear?

Do you know of any reason why your periods have stopped?

Is there any chance that you might be pregnant?

I would now like to ask you both some questions about puberty, because it may be that Anne is just a late starter.

To the mother

At what age did you go through puberty?

At what age did you have your growth spurt?

At what age did you start your periods?

Is there anyone else in your family who was a late starter?

To Anne

Have you any hair in your armpits? — If so, when did you first notice this?

When did you first notice pubic hair?

Have your breasts started to develop — If so, when did that happen?

Are you an athlete or a 'fitness fanatic'?

Do you have any other symptoms?

How is your appetite?

Is your weight steady?

Have you had any illnesses in the recent past?

Have you noticed an increasing growth of hair on your face and arms?

Has there been any discharge of milk from your breasts?

Have you noticed a milk scab on your nipples or on your bra?

SCOFF questionnaire

Do you make yourself Sick because you feel uncomfortably full?

Do you worry that you have lost Control over how much you eat?

Have you recently lost more than One stone in a 3-month period?

Do you believe yourself to be Fat when others say you are thin?

Would you say that Food dominates your life?

Mrs Slater, a 60-year-old lady, has been told by her friends that she is becoming jaundiced. Please ask her some questions.

Jaundice (yellow pigmentation of the skin and sclerae) is the clinical manifestation of hyperbilirubinaemia. It is useful to remember that carotenaemia, caused by the ingestion and absorption of large amounts of carotene (found in carrots), does not cause scleral pigmentation. The causes of jaundice are traditionally divided into *prehepatic*, *hepatocellular*, and *obstructive*.

Prehepatic jaundice

- Haemolysis (intravascular and extravascular)
- Ineffective erythropoiesis — thalassaemia major, megaloblastic anaemia
- Impaired conjugation — Gilbert's syndrome, drugs (e.g. chloramphenicol), sepsis

Hepatocellular jaundice

- Viral hepatitis
- Drug-induced cholestasis (e.g. chlorpromazine, androgens)
- Alcoholic liver disease
- Biliary cirrhosis (primary or secondary)

Extrahepatic defects

- Intraductal obstruction — gall stones, malignancy (ampullary carcinoma, cholangiocarcinoma), sclerosing cholangitis, biliary malformations (strictures, atresia), infection
- Biliary tract compression — pancreatic cancer, lymph node enlargement at the porta hepatis

History

When evaluating this 60-year-old patient with jaundice you should start by determining the *duration* of the jaundice and then proceed to ask about any *associated symptoms* such as abdominal pain, pruritus, fever or a change in appetite, weight or bowel habit. An assessment of *risk factors* is important (blood transfusion, intravenous drug abuse, travel overseas, alcohol) as is a *drug history*. The most important cause to be excluded in this patient is an underlying malignancy.

Questions

When did your friends first notice that you had turned yellow?

Has the yellowness become deeper with time?

Has this ever happened before?

Have your motions changed colour?

For example, have they become pale?

Have you noticed any change in the colour of your urine?

Have you had a recent flu-like illness?

Do you get unexplained itching?

Have you had any sweats or rigors?

Do you get any abdominal pain?

Have you lost any weight? How much?

Do you have any other medical problem?

Are you taking any medication?

Do you drink any alcohol? If so, how much in a week?

Have you been abroad recently?

Have you had any blood transfusions in the past?

Have you had any operations recently?

Are you married or in a stable relationship?

If not, are you sexually active?

Do you take any recreational drugs? (*unlikely in a 60-year-old lady*)

Has anyone in your family ever had jaundice?

Mr Miller is a 30-year-old gentleman referred by his GP. He presented to her with generalized lymphadenopathy that has been present for the past 3 weeks. Please take a history to identify a possible cause.

Generalized lymphadenopathy can be caused by systemic infections, malignancies, immunological reactions or by a number of lymphadenopathy syndromes.

Systemic infections

- Viral infections — infectious hepatitis, infectious mononucleosis syndromes (Epstein–Barr virus, cytomegalovirus), AIDS, rubella
- Bacterial infections — tuberculosis, brucellosis, cat-scratch fever, secondary syphilis
- Parasitic — toxoplasmosis

Immunological diseases

- Drug reactions — phenytoin, hydralazine, allopurinol, silicone implants
- Angioimmunoblastic lymphadenopathy
- Autoimmune disorders — rheumatoid arthritis, Sjögren's syndrome, SLE

Malignancy

- Non-Hodgkin's lymphoma
- Hodgkin's disease
- Acute lymphoblastic leukaemia
- Chronic lymphocytic leukaemia
- Metastatic carcinoma

Other causes

- Hyperthyroidism
- Sarcoidosis
- Amyloidosis
- Familial Mediterranean fever
- Mucocutaneous lymph node syndrome

History

As this patient has presented with a 3-week history of generalized lymphadenopathy an *infectious cause* or a *lymphoma* are the most likely causes. You should elicit a detailed history to identify possible infection and enquire specifically about associated symptoms (fever, night sweats and weight loss). Ask questions about risk factors for HIV infection, drug history, travel history, and contact with pets.

Questions

When did you first notice these lumps?

Did they appear suddenly or gradually? In other words, were you all right one day and the next day you noticed these lumps?

Did they start in only one place? — If so, where exactly?

Have they increased or decreased in size or remained the same?

Are they painful or tender to touch?

Have you had any flu-like symptoms recently?

Any sore throats?

Do you suffer from frequent infections?

Do you bruise easily or have you noticed any skin rashes?

Have you lost any weight? If so, how much?

How much did you weigh in the past compared with now?

Have you had any night sweats?

Have you had any high temperatures or rigors recently?

Do you have any other illnesses?

Are you on any medication?

Occasionally enlargement of these lymph nodes may be caused by unusual viral infections such as HIV, the virus that causes

AIDS. Are you aware of any risk factors that you may have been exposed to for HIV infection, such as haemophilia, blood transfusions, intravenous drug use, or unprotected sex?

Have you been abroad recently?

Have you had TB before or have you been in contact with anybody with TB recently?

Mr Grant is a 25-year-old man with a severe headache of 1 hour's duration. Please take a history from him.

The short duration of the headache suggests that the onset might have been sudden and your initial differential diagnosis should include the following four conditions:

- Subarachnoid haemorrhage
- Thunderclap headache
- Migraine
- Acute meningitis

Thunderclap headache is a sudden, severe, 'exploding' pain that involves the entire head and resolves gradually over hours. It is of sudden onset, as in subarachnoid haemorrhage, from which it is often indistinguishable, but the investigations in most cases do not show any vascular lesion.

History

Your initial enquiry will have to establish if the headache was of sudden onset and, if so, which one of these conditions is the most likely cause. If the onset was not rapid then you will have to consider other causes such as *tension headache*. The patient with a *subarachnoid haemorrhage* or a *thunderclap headache* may tell you that he felt as if a brick hit his head. *Migraine* may be preceded by a prodromal phase during which the patient may see flashing lights with a zigzag pattern. If the patient describes this he should be asked more questions about the duration of this phase and if he experiences any other symptoms with it. The hemicrania of migraine, unlike that caused by an intracranial vascular malformation, will occasionally change sides although it may favour one side. He should also be asked if there is anything that brings on these headaches and anything that relieves them.

Questions

How did your headache start — was it sudden or has it been building up gradually?

If sudden — Was it abrupt — one second you were all right and the next second you had a headache?

Did you have any symptoms before the headache or any premonition that you were going to get it?

Have you had any similar episodes in the past?

If yes — How often do you get it?

Do you go three to six months or only a month without it?

Is the headache only on one side or on both sides of your head?

If one-sided — Does it always start on that side or does it sometimes start on the other side?

Do you have any other symptoms such as nausea, a stiff neck, or a dislike of bright light?

Is there anything such as coughing, straining, or standing, that aggravates your headache and is there anything that eases it?

Is there any family history of similar headaches? (*suggestive of migraine*)

Do any of your close relatives get headaches?

John is a 1-year-old baby and his mother is worried because of his screaming attacks during which he draws up his legs. Please take a history from his mother.

Screaming attacks associated with curling up of the legs suggest colicky pain in the abdomen in an infant of this age. Three conditions merit consideration and the mother should be questioned carefully so that the first of these is not missed:

- Intussusception
- Acute gastroenteritis
- Urinary tract infection

History

In *intussusception* screaming attacks recur every 15–20 minutes and last for 2–4 minutes. In *gastroenteritis* the stools are watery, voluminous, and smelly. In intussusception, the stools will be scanty and may have a currant-jelly appearance caused by oozing of blood from the congested intussusceptum. Screaming attacks may also occur in association with a *urinary tract infection* as micturition may be frequent and painful (and the urine usually smelly).

Questions

How often does John have these screaming attacks?

How long does each attack last for?

Does his colour change during these?

Does he turn pale? (*intussusception*)

Has he been vomiting? (*intussusception, gastroenteritis*)

Has he passed any stools?

Has he had diarrhoea?

How many motions has he had today?

What is the colour of his stools?

Do the attacks occur only during micturition?

Does his urine smell?

Mr Thomas is a 65-year-old man who presented to his GP with a 1-month history of fresh bleeding from his back passage. Please take a history.

A history of fresh bleeding suggests that the responsible lesion is probably in the *lower* intestinal tract and you should consider:

- Haemorrhoids
- Anal fissure
- Colitis — Crohn's disease, ulcerative, infective, ischaemic, post-radiation
- Polyps
- Carcinoma (large bowel)
- Diverticular disease
- Angiodysplasia of the colon
- Meckel's diverticulum
- Drugs (e.g. warfarin)

History

It is important to know if the blood loss is separate from, or mixed in with, the stools, as this will determine whether the source is anorectal or in the large bowel.

Questions

Have you noticed any blood on the surface of the stools or has the toilet paper been blood stained?

Does the blood come before, with, or after the stools?

Do you also pass any mucus?

Have you had this before?

Do you have any pain when you open your bowels? (*anal fissure*)
Has there been any change in your bowel habit?
Have you lost any weight, and how is your appetite?
Have you been unwell or had a fever recently? (*infective*)
Have you been abroad recently? (*infective*)
Do you have any other medical problems?
Are you on any medication?

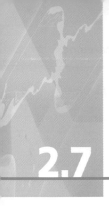

Mr Jackson is a 60-year-old man. He has noticed blood in his urine. Take a history regarding this complaint.

It is worth recalling some of the possible causes of haematuria before considering your line of questioning:

- Urinary tract infection
- Calculi
- Prostatitis
- Drugs — analgesic nephropathy due to non-steroidal anti-inflammatory drugs (NSAIDs), warfarin
- Trauma
- Tumours (benign and malignant)
- Tuberculosis
- Focal glomerulonephritis
- Sickle cell disorders
- IgA nephropathy

History

It is important to find out whether the blood comes at the beginning, during, or at the end of micturition. *Initial haematuria* is suggestive of prostatic or urethral causes. Reddish urine throughout the stream (*total haematuria*) indicates that blood has mixed with urine in the bladder, suggesting the kidney, ureter, or bladder as the source of haemorrhage. *Painless haematuria* is suggestive of a neoplasm, coagulopathy (e.g. caused by warfarin), glomerulonephritis or tuberculosis. *Painful haematuria* is suggestive of calculi, urinary tract infection, or trauma. *Fever and rigors* are suggestive of an infection. Sickle cell disease is possible in a patient of Afro-Caribbean origin. *Weight loss* would be suggestive of a malignancy or chronic infection.

Questions

Do you pass blood at the beginning or at the end of passing water, or is it occurring throughout the stream?

Do you have pain or a burning sensation while passing urine?

Do you get any spasms of pain in your tummy?

Have you felt hot or feverish?

Do you get shivery with the fever?

Does your urine smell?

How is your appetite?

Have you lost any weight?

Have you had any injuries recently?

Are you on any medication? (*warfarin, NSAIDs*)

Do you have any other medical problems? (*e.g. sickle cell disease, diabetes mellitus*)

Mrs Lewis is a 70-year-old diabetic lady presenting with pain and swelling in the left knee. Ask her some questions to arrive at a diagnosis.

The differential diagnosis of monoarticular (single joint) involvement of the knee joint with pain and an effusion (clear or purulent) is:

- Infection (septic arthritis)
- Trauma
- Osteoarthrosis
- Crystalline arthropathy — gout, pseudogout (chondrocalcinosis)

History

Infection is a strong possibility because this lady is a diabetic. *Pseudogout* also occurs more commonly in this age group, particularly when there is an associated medical condition such as diabetes mellitus, hyperparathyroidism, haemochromatosis, hypothyroidism or Wilson's disease.

Septic arthritis must be excluded because it can progress to septicaemia (ask about any constitutional symptoms such as fever, malaise, headache, etc.) and it will require specific antibiotic treatment for 6 weeks. *Osteoarthrosis* may cause an effusion in one knee but of course there would be a past history of joint disease. Similarly, there will be a positive history of joint problems if she has sustained an *injury* to her knee or if she has had rheumatoid arthritis.

In pseudogout the knee is commonly the site of inflammation as a result of calcium pyrophosphate crystal deposition. The onset may be acute in both gout and pseudogout and the pain may be unbearable. Both these conditions have a familial tendency. Though it can recur, septic arthritis (also painful) is usually a first event; pseudogout is usually a recurrent condition.

Questions

How long has the knee been swollen?

Has it been getting worse?

Have you had a temperature or felt unwell?

Are there any other joints involved?

Has the joint been hot and red?

Have you injured your knee recently?

Has this joint been swollen before?

Do you have any other serious medical conditions?

Mr Munro, a 25-year-old gentleman, is brought to Casualty after what appears to have been an epileptic fit at home. Please take a history.

An *epileptic seizure* is a convulsion or transient abnormal event experienced by a patient caused by a paroxysmal discharge of cortical neurones. *Epilepsy* is the continuing tendency to have such seizures (even if there are long intervals between episodes). A generalized convulsion or *grand mal* fit is the most common type of seizure. It is a common condition and 2–3% of the population have two or more fits during their lives. Although in most cases no specific cause of epilepsy is uncovered, you should bear in mind the possible aetiological and precipitating factors:

- Family history (30% have a positive history of fits in a first-degree relative)
- History of trauma or surgery to the head
- History of febrile convulsions in infancy
- Intracranial mass lesions affecting the cerebral cortex
- Stroke (cerebral infarction)
- Drugs (phenothiazines, monoamine oxidase inhibitors, tricyclic antidepressants, amphetamines), drug withdrawal (anticonvulsants, benzodiazepines), chronic alcohol abuse
- Infections — encephalitis, tuberculous meningitis, cerebral abscess, neurosyphilis
- Metabolic abnormalities — hypocalcaemia, hypoglycaemia, hyponatraemia, acute hypoxia
- Flashing strobe lighting or flickering TV screens (photosensitivity)

History

First you have to establish whether or not this event was an epileptic fit and then probe into any possible causative factors. It is always important to get a full account of the fit from both the patient and, if possible, a witness. If the history *is* suggestive of an epileptic fit ask appropriate questions to identify the type. Next, try to identify any aetiological factors from the history. The occupational history may be important for future management.

Questions

Tell me what actually happened at home?

To the witness:

Did he have any shaking of the limbs?
Did it start in a particular part of the body?
Did the shaking involve one side of the body or both sides?
Did he lose consciousness?

To the patient:

Did you 'wet yourself' during the fit?
Did you bite your tongue?
Did you fall and injure yourself?
When you came round did you know where you were?
How did you feel afterwards?
Have you had any injuries recently?
Have you had any headaches recently?
Do you have any problems with your vision?
Have you felt uncomfortable with bright light recently?
Do you have any other medical problems?
Have you had fits before?

History of previous fits:

When was the first fit and how often do they occur?

Do they occur during the day or only at night?

Are you on any medication?

If yes — Had you taken your usual tablets today?

What investigations have you had?

Does anyone in your family have epilepsy?

What is your occupation?

Mrs Saunders is a 60-year-old lady presenting with an ulcer over the lateral malleolus of her right ankle. Ask her some questions to help you to identify the underlying cause.

The most likely cause of an ulcer over the lateral malleolus in this patient would be an infarctive ulcer which characteristically affects the malleoli in hypertensive and diabetic subjects. However, you should also consider other possibilities:

- Venous insufficiency (stasis ulcer) — thrombosis, varicose veins, passive venous congestion, venous obstruction
- Arterial insufficiency (anterior or lower lateral leg, painful with cold blue feet)
  - atherosclerosis obliterans (usually affects toes which become gangrenous)
  - Buerger's disease (occurs predominantly in young, male smokers)
- Pressure sore (decubitus ulcer)
- Vasculitis — rheumatoid arthritis, systemic lupus erythematosus, pyoderma gangrenosum
- Infection — post-cellulitis, TB, leprosy
- Tumour — squamous cell/basal cell carcinoma, Kaposi's sarcoma
- Haematological — sickle cell, thalassaemia, paroxysmal nocturnal haemoglobinuria
- Neuropathic — diabetes, tabes, leprosy, syringomyelia
- Trauma
- Dermatitis artefacta (i.e. self-inflicted)

In general, leg ulcers occur in the older population. *Venous insufficiency, arterial insufficiency, pressure sores* and *diabetes* are the main causes.

Venous ulcers

Venous ulcers are confined to the lower leg and are often post-thrombotic. Incompetent valves in the veins cause an increase in hydrostatic pressure and capillary blood pressure. Plasma leaks under pressure leading to perivascular fibrin deposition and a decrease in oxygen supply. Skin nutrition is affected which leads to ischaemia and eventual ulceration.

Venous ulcers around or just above the ankle are often associated with:

- hyperpigmentation due to haemosiderin deposition from red cell extravasation
- dermatitis and excoriation from itching
- secondary infection

Arterial ulcers

Arterial ulcers (particularly those due to atherosclerosis) usually occur on the legs but may occasionally occur on the feet. They may accompany venous hypertension, especially in the elderly.

Associated features:

- Cold atrophic skin with loss of hair
- Poor peripheral pulses
- History of claudication
- Ulcer may have a punched-out appearance
- Doppler studies may confirm arterial insufficiency

Pressure sores

Decubitus ulcers, or pressure sores, form as a result of skin ischaemia from prolonged pressure over a bony point in a patient who is unable to turn regularly. They often occur over the sacrum, hip or heel. The majority of them occur in hospital and often on orthopaedic wards. About three-quarters of patients with very deep ulcers will not survive.

Predisposing factors include:

- Old age
- Immobility (especially bedridden patients)
- Long periods spent on hospital trolleys in Casualty departments
- Post-operative period

- Altered sensation of the skin
- Poor circulation
- Poor tissue nutrition
- Diabetes mellitus
- Anaemia
- Dehydration
- Oedema
- Urinary incontinence

History

As stated above, the scenario given suggests that this patient has an infarctive or *Martorell's ulcer* which characteristically affects the lower legs of hypertensive patients (posterolaterally or medially), especially in those who also have diabetes. These ulcers are caused by avascular necrosis of the skin, and develop rapidly with severe pain. These considerations should be borne in mind when asking questions, and other possible diagnoses should not be overlooked. Other vascular causes of a leg ulcer should be explored as they form the most important differential diagnosis in this patient.

The history should identify appropriate aetiological factors. Diabetics are more at risk of infection and arterial disease. Recent cellulitis may lead to ulceration of the leg. Chronic dependent swelling can predispose to ulceration. Intermittent claudication would suggest an arterial, atherosclerotic ulcer. Rheumatoid arthritis and inflammatory bowel disease may be associated with pyoderma gangrenosum.

Questions

Tell me how the ulcer started — Did it develop within a day or more gradually?

How long have you had the ulcer?

Did you have any complaints before the ulcer appeared?

Was there any previous discoloration of the skin?

Have you had any redness or inflammation of the surrounding skin recently?

Does it produce any discharge? — If so, what colour and in what quantity?

Do you feel any pain? (*absence of pain suggests that there may be a neuropathic element*)

Do you have varicose veins?

Are you a diabetic?

Do you have high blood pressure?

Do you smoke?

Do you sit for very long periods of time?

Has the affected leg been lying on its side for a long time?

Have you had any injury to the leg recently?

Do you get any cramp-like pains in your calves when you walk which get better when you rest?

Have you got any problems with your joints or your bowels?

Do you have any other medical problems?

Mr Taylor is a 45-year-old bus driver. He has vomited blood on two occasions in the past week. Take a history in order to arrive at a diagnosis.

The causes of *upper gastrointestinal haemorrhage* are:

- Chronic peptic ulceration — gastric and duodenal ulcers (50%)
- Acute gastric ulcers and erosions (20%)
- Mallory–Weiss syndrome (5–10%)
- Varices (5–10%)
- Reflux oesophagitis (5%)
- Drugs (may be contributory in many cases) — aspirin, NSAIDs, anticoagulants
- Alcohol (in excessive quantities)
- Gastric cancer (uncommon)
- Other rarer causes — hereditary haemorrhagic telangiectasia (Osler–Weber–Rendu syndrome), pseudoxanthoma elasticum, blood dyscrasias

History

In a 45-year-old man nonmalignant causes are more likely. Small haemorrhages are more serious in older age. Excessive vomiting can cause an oesophageal tear (Mallory–Weiss syndrome). The presence of melaena would support the diagnosis of a significant upper gastrointestinal haemorrhage. An underlying history of peptic ulcer disease can be elicited in many patients. Drug-induced gastritis is an important cause of gastrointestinal haemorrhage but other risk factors for peptic ulcer disease, including smoking, alcohol, and stress should be explored. An estimate of alcohol consumption should be obtained (?oesophageal varices).

Questions

Would you like to tell me about your vomiting and how it started?

How much blood did you vomit each time?

Was it an eggcupful, a cupful or more?

What was its colour?

Has this happened before?

Have you had any vomiting before these two episodes?

Have you passed any blood or black motions?

Have you had any indigestion in the past?

Have you been told that you have an ulcer in your stomach?

Do you have a hiatus hernia?

Have you had heartburn, pain or discomfort in your stomach?

Do you have any other medical problems?

Are you on any medication? (*e.g. anti-ulcer drugs, aspirin, NSAIDs, anticoagulants*)

Do you smoke? — If so, how much?

Do you drink alcohol — If so, how much do you drink and how long have you been drinking that amount?

Have you lost your appetite?

Have you lost any weight?

Mrs Brown is a 36-year-old lady with pain in the right iliac fossa. Please take a history.

There are acute and chronic causes for pain in the right iliac fossa.

Acute causes

- Surgical emergencies — acute appendicitis, intestinal obstruction, ureteric colic, perforated peptic ulcer, acute cholecystitis, bowel infarction
- Obstetric emergency — ectopic pregnancy
- Gynaecological causes — e.g. twisted ovarian cyst
- Other causes — acute pyelonephritis, enterocolitis, intra-abdominal haemorrhage, acute intermittent porphyria

Chronic causes

- Salpingitis
- Regional ileitis
- Appendicular abscess
- Ileocaecal tuberculosis
- Mittelschmerz (dysmenorrhoea intermenstrualis)
- Caecal carcinoma

History

The history of *onset* and the *duration* of the pain are crucial to differentiate acute from chronic causes of right iliac fossa pain. The *type* of pain also gives a clue about the underlying cause (constant pain: may indicate nonobstructive appendicitis, ectopic pregnancy, or salpingitis; colicky pain: occurs in obstructive appendicitis, intestinal obstruction, or ureteric colic).

The following *features of the pain* are important and should be explored through appropriate questions.

Initial site

- Umbilical area — appendicitis, intestinal obstruction
- Epigastrium — perforated peptic ulcer, appendicitis
- Right hypochondrium — acute cholecystitis
- Right iliac fossa — ectopic pregnancy
- Loin — pyelonephritis, ureteric colic, twisted ovarian cyst

Radiation

- Loin to groin — ureteric colic
- Low down — salpingitis

Aggravating factors

- On coughing — appendicitis (but not with ureteric colic)
- On rolling — twisted ovarian cyst

Associated symptoms

- Nausea and vomiting — appendicitis, intestinal obstruction
- Diarrhoea — enterocolitis, Crohn's disease
- Weight loss — cancer, tuberculosis
- Menstrual problems — pelvic inflammatory disease

Questions

Tell me about your pain — when and where did it start?

How long have you had this pain?

What does it feel like?

Is it a constant or a colicky pain?

Does the pain go anywhere else?

Does anything that you do make the pain worse?

Have you felt sick or actually been sick?

Have you passed any blood or mucus?

Have you missed any periods? (*ectopic pregnancy*)

Have you had any other problems with your periods recently? (*salpingitis*)

Have you had any discharge down below?

Have you had any tummy pains before? (*dyspepsia, mittelschmerz*)

Have you had diarrhoea or constipation recently?

How is your appetite?

Have you lost any weight?

Have you had any fevers or night sweats recently?

Do you have any other medical problems?

Are you on any medication?

Mr Smith is a 65-year-old man presenting with weight loss which has occurred over the past few months. Ask him some questions.

Unintended weight loss is a nonspecific, but serious, symptom. A clinically useful classification of the many possible causes (and associated symptoms) is given below.

Loss of weight in spite of increased food intake

- Diabetes mellitus (with polyphagia, polyuria, and polydipsia)
- Thyrotoxicosis (with polyphagia, irritability, heat intolerance, and diarrhoea)
- Malabsorption states (with polyphagia, diarrhoea, and intolerance to particular foods)

Loss of weight with decreased food intake

- Malignancy (with change in bowel habit, abdominal pain, blood in the stools, lumps, fevers, and night sweats)
- Chronic infections — tuberculosis (with fevers, night sweats, and history of contact)
- Chronic system failure — chronic obstructive airways disease, congestive cardiac failure, chronic renal failure, chronic liver disease
- Mental disorders — depression
- Endocrine insufficiency — adrenal failure (with weakness, tiredness, pigmentation, and postural hypotension), panhypopituitarism (with loss of libido, amenorrhoea, impotence, tiredness, pallor, and hair loss)

History

When taking a history from a patient with weight loss you should make sure first that the patient is not consciously dieting!

Establish if there is loss of appetite leading to reduced food intake. In a 65-year-old man with reduced appetite, *malignancy* should be on top of the list. However, *depression, diabetes mellitus* and *chronic system failure* should be excluded.

Questions

Please tell me how you discovered that you had lost weight?

Are you in the habit of weighing yourself?

When did you last weigh yourself?

What is your weight now? How much weight have you lost? (*>10% weight loss is significant*)

How is your appetite?

Has there been any alteration in your eating habits?

If he admits to losing his appetite:

Has there been any change in your bowel habit recently?

Have you had any abdominal pains?

Have you noticed any blood in your stools?

Have you felt any lumps?

Do you have any long-standing medical problems?

Have you had any fevers or night sweats recently?

Have you been abroad recently?

Have you felt low or depressed lately?

If he describes an increase in appetite:

Do you eat more than you used to?

Do you feel excessively thirsty? (*diabetes mellitus*)

How much have you been drinking?

Do you pass a lot of water? (*diabetes mellitus*)

Have you felt tremulous, sweaty or anxious recently? (*thyrotoxicosis*)

Do you prefer cold or warm weather?

Have you had loose stools?

Has there been any difficulty flushing away your stool in the toilet? (*steatorrhoea*)

Is there any particular food that causes any problems?

Mr White, a 70-year-old man, presents with a 6-month history of hesitancy and poor urinary stream. Please take a history.

History

Hesitancy and poor urinary stream suggest bladder outflow obstruction. In a 70-year-old man prostatic enlargement, due to *benign prostatic hyperplasia* or *prostatic cancer,* is the most likely cause of the obstructive symptoms. Questions about other urinary symptoms (frequency, urgency, nocturia, terminal dribbling, incontinence) should be asked. Chronic obstruction of the urinary tract may lead to *renal insufficiency* and you should ask questions to assess this possibility.

Questions

I understand you are having trouble with your waterworks. Would you please describe it to me?

Do you pass water frequently?

How often do you pass water?

Do you have to get up at night to pass water? (*nocturia*)

Do you have the urge to pass water all the time?

Do you have a sense of incomplete emptying of your bladder after you have been to the toilet?

Can you make a good stream?

Do you dribble at the end? (*terminal dribbling*)

Do you pass small amounts more frequently?

Do you have any scalding or burning or pain when passing water?

Can you hold your water or do you have to rush to the nearest toilet?

Have you noticed any blood in your water recently?

Do you get frequent urinary infections? (*due to urinary retention or bladder calculus*)

Do you have any pain anywhere? (*back pain suggests prostate cancer; loin pain suggests hydronephrosis*)

Have you lost any weight?

How is your appetite? (*cancer, renal failure*)

Mr Johnson is a 25-year-old man who says he is hearing voices. They terrify him. Please take a history.

Auditory hallucinations (hearing voices without any obvious source) are most common in schizophrenic states but they also occur in toxic confusional conditions, involutional melancholia and in the senile dementias. The young age of this patient would exclude the last two conditions, and the mention of hallucinations alone would make toxic confusion unlikely. However, one would have to ask a few questions to test his memory and orientation to explore this diagnosis (see p. 89). This scenario suggests *schizophrenia*, as the main possibility, in which cognitive function is usually intact in the early stages. The voices are usually localized as coming from the head or some part of the body (very typical of schizophrenia), but may appear to come from outside. Important features that are considered diagnostic of schizophrenia are the symptoms known as *Schneider's first-rank symptoms*.

Schneider's first-rank symptoms of schizophrenia

- Auditory hallucinations — the hearing of voices repeating the patient's thoughts out loud and/or discussing the patient in the third person and/or giving a running commentary on the patient's behaviour
- Thought insertion — the patient's belief that external thoughts are being inserted into his mind by an external or alien agency
- Thought withdrawal — the patient's belief that his thoughts are being removed by an external power
- Thought broadcasting — the patient's belief that his thoughts are being 'read' by someone, as if they were being broadcast

- External control of feelings, impulses and actions — the patient's feeling that his free will has been removed and that he is being controlled by an external agency
- Somatic passivity — the patient's belief that he is a passive recipient of somatic (bodily) sensations from an external agency
- Delusional perception — a delusional misrepresentation of a real perception (For example, the patient, when he sees someone coming towards him, may believe that he is a general and that the man coming up to him is his adjutant.)

The patient may also have *tactile hallucinations* and feel sensations of intense cold, heat, or drizzling. Some schizophrenic patients feel that their body, or a part of it, has changed in size or weight. *Olfactory hallucinations* with an unpleasant character may be present in schizophrenia. Other characteristic features are *persistent delusions* (of a religious or political identity or of possession of superhuman powers), *persistent hallucinations* (half-formed delusions without clear affective content, or belief in ideas which are demonstrably false), *breaks or interpolations in the train of thought, neologisms* (new words constructed by the patient or everyday words used in a special way), and *catatonic behaviour* (stupor, akinesia, excitement, posturing, etc.). Schizophrenic patients do not cope well with emotional intensity of any kind and tend to live within a narrow range of emotional and environmental stimulation. The first attack of schizophrenia may be precipitated by such stresses as leaving home to go to college or to join the army, or the loss of a girlfriend or of a job.

History

It is clear from the above that this patient should be asked questions not only about the voices he is hearing but also about his personal, social, family, and environmental circumstances. As in any psychiatric interview, it is important to maintain a relaxed atmosphere, to be nonjudgemental about his symptoms, and to explore the patient's own perception of his illness. Your line of questioning will depend to some extent on the patient's answers to your initial questions.

Questions

Why do you think you were referred here?

Do you have any idea about what is wrong with you?

About these voices — are they constant or do they come and go?

Can you make out what is being said or are they just sounds?

Do you think that someone else is trying to influence you? — Who?

Are they talking about you or repeating your thoughts?

Is someone saying something in anticipation of what you had thought?

Do you feel in full control of yourself or is someone influencing your actions?

Do you feel any other sensations in your body?

Have you had any other problems recently?

What is your occupation?

Have you had the same job for a while?

Do you have any hobbies?

Do you live with your parents or by yourself?

How do you get on with your friends and your family?

Is there any history of a 'nervous' disease in your extended family?

Sam is a 6-month-old baby boy sent up to the clinic by the GP with 'failure to thrive'. Ask his anxious mother some relevant questions in an effort to uncover a possible underlying cause.

Failure to thrive, or wasting, during the first year of an infant's life, also known as *marasmus*, results from an inadequate or improper feeding regime in the Western world; simple starvation due to unavailability of food is a common cause in many other parts of the world. The marasmic infant's weight lies below the third centile on growth charts. The commonest causes are *mismanagement of feeding, infections,* and *malabsorption* although a wide variety of conditions must be considered in the differential diagnosis.

Causes of marasmus

1. *Underfeeding.* An improper or disturbed feeding regime is the commonest cause, though there may be associated emotional deprivation, frank neglect, or even child abuse. The mother may be careless with the preparation of feeds, may show an abnormal aloofness during feeding, or may not respond to the emotional needs of the baby, either because the pregnancy was unwanted or because the baby was of the 'wrong' sex.
2. *Infections.* Infantile gastroenteritis is a common problem but other recurrent or chronic infections such as bronchopneumonia, osteomyelitis, pyelonephritis, skin infections and, rarely, tuberculosis may cause marasmus.
3. *Congenital structural abnormalities.* Cyanotic and acyanotic cardiac anomalies, hydrocephalus, renal anomalies (bladder-neck obstruction, ureteric reflux, hydronephrosis, renal hypoplasia), pyloric stenosis, atresia of the bile ducts,

Hirschsprung's disease, and deformities of the palate and jaws which interfere with feeding may all cause marasmus.

4. *Cystic fibrosis.*   Deficient nutrition is caused by intestinal malabsorption, compounded by the invariable occurrence of episodes of lung sepsis.

5. *Metabolic disorders.*   These include intestinal malabsorption due to cow's milk protein (lactose) intolerance, hyperchloraemic renal acidosis, Fanconi syndrome, nephrogenic diabetes insipidus and galactosaemia.

6. *Coeliac disease.*   Although this condition seldom occurs before the second year of life, early introduction of gluten-containing cereals may lead to an earlier onset of malabsorption.

7. *Hypothalamic tumour.*   This syndrome of emaciation associated with a diencephalic tumour is diagnosed after the more usual causes have been excluded. Characteristic features are emaciation (although the length is usually above average) and marked hyperactivity with incongruous euphoria.

History

The correct diagnosis of marasmus requires strict adherence to the basic principles of history-taking. The first requirement is to establish that Sam *is* underweight and small compared with other infants of his age and sex. Your enquiry should then be extended to assess the mother's health before and during the pregnancy and her psychological state after the delivery. There may be a history of rubella during the first trimester or of placental insufficiency during the last trimester. Feeding should be explored in detail and questions should be asked about the type of feeds, the times they are given, and if the infant is satisfied after each feed. The mother should be asked delicately if she feels emotionally involved when she feeds Sam.

A careful enquiry will elicit whether Sam is underfed and passes 'starvation stools' (dark green mucoid stains on the nappy) or has gastroenteritis and passes the large, watery, green stools of infection. In cystic fibrosis the stools may be described as being greasy and foul smelling and there may be a history of a spasmodic cough. The exertion of feeding results in breathlessness in congestive cardiac failure and the mother may complain that the baby 'gets tired' halfway through his feeds. You should ask if the infant has had any attacks of projectile vomiting (pyloric stenosis) or has attacks of abdominal colic in which he draws his legs up (urinary infection). The following questions may have to be extended in a particular direction, depending on the answers given.

Questions

Do you think that Sam is small for his age and sex?

Have you kept a record of his weight and height? — If so, may I please have a look at it?

Are you still breast- or bottle-feeding him or have you weaned him off milk feeds?

When did you start weaning him off milk feeds?

Do you prepare his feeds according to the manufacturer's instructions?

Have you introduced any cereals in his feeds?

Does he complete his feeds satisfactorily or does he get tired?

Do you have some 'baby talk' with him before and during feeding?

What colour are his stools?

Are they bulky, scanty or watery?

How are his waterworks? Does he scream or draw up his legs when he passes water?

Does he vomit after feeding?

How was your health during and after the pregnancy?

Did you have regular antenatal check ups?

Did you deliver at full term or was the pregnancy induced earlier for any reason?

Did you have any postnatal 'blues'?

What was his birth weight?

Mr James is a 45-year-old man who was found to have glycosuria at a routine insurance examination. His GP has sent him to you for evaluation. Ask him some relevant questions.

This is not an unusual scenario as a patient with glycosuria detected on routine dipstick testing may or may not have any symptoms of *diabetes mellitus*. The only other explanation for this finding is *renal glycosuria* in which there is a low renal threshold for glucose and it is passed in the urine at normal plasma glucose levels. Although the history may give some useful clues about the likelihood of diabetes mellitus, the ultimate diagnosis will depend on the blood glucose levels.

Biochemical diagnosis of diabetes mellitus

Random glucose levels
Diabetes mellitus is likely if random testing shows:

Venous plasma glucose	≥11.1 mmol/L
Capillary plasma glucose	≥12.2 mmol/L
Venous whole blood glucose	≥10.0 mmol/L
Capillary whole blood glucose	≥11.1 mmol/L

Fasting glucose levels
Diabetes mellitus is likely if fasting levels are:

Venous plasma glucose	≥7.0 mmol/ L
Capillary plasma glucose	≥7.0 mmol/ L
Venous whole blood glucose	≥6.1 mmol/ L
Capillary whole blood glucose	≥6.1 mmol/ L

Glucose tolerance test

If the random and fasting glucose levels are borderline a formal 75 g oral glucose tolerance test is required. The diagnosis is established if 2-hour levels are:

Venous plasma glucose	≥ 11.1 mmol/L
Capillary plasma glucose	≥ 12.2 mmol/L
Venous whole blood glucose	≥ 10.0 mmol/L
Capillary whole blood glucose	≥ 11.1 mmol/L

History

Although this short history should concentrate on the manifestations of diabetes mellitus and its complications, the patient should also be asked if he has had glycosuria in the past, for example, at a previous routine test. He may also have noticed white spots on his shoes — after micturition a few droplets may fall on the shoes which dry to white spots if the urine contains sugar. A diagnosis of renal glycosuria is likely if the patient has had glycosuria for a long time without any symptoms of diabetes mellitus.

Questions

Were you surprised when you were told that you have sugar in your urine? *(He won't be if he has been found to have glycosuria in the past.)*

Have you had a similar check-up in the past? — If so, did they make any comments?

Has anyone had occasion to test your urine in the past? — If so, with what results?

Have you ever seen unexplained white spots on your shoes?

Has there been any change in your eating and drinking habits?

Do you have excessive thirst and drink a lot of fluids?

Do you pass a lot of water?

What is your appetite like?

Is your weight steady or have you lost or gained any weight?

Have you had any infections recently?

Have you had any blurring of vision?

Have you experienced any numbness or tingling in your hands and feet?

Has anyone among your close relatives had diabetes mellitus?

Mrs Green, a 69-year-old lady, presents with a 3-month history of fatigue and a 2-day history of constant pain in the left iliac fossa. She looks pale and breathless. Please take a history.

The question contains a few clues which should allow the candidate to narrow down the number of possible diagnoses. The history is clearly one of insidious onset, at first gradually progressive but now presenting with acute symptoms. The pallor and breathlessness are most likely to be due to anaemia, a clue that this lady has had chronic blood loss from the gut. The constant pain of two days' duration does not, of course, exclude episodes of pain in the past and the patient may have other symptoms related to her bowels, such as diarrhoea, constipation, or the passage of black stools.

While the details given suggest that the pathology is most likely to be found in the bowel, you must not forget the possibility that she may have a systemic illness (e.g. pernicious anaemia, subacute endocarditis, myeloproliferative disorder) and that the abdominal pain may or may not be related to the main problem.

You should consider the following differential diagnoses:

- Bowel malignancy
- Diverticular disease
- Inflammatory bowel disease
- Anaemia from any other cause
- Hypothyroidism with constipation

History

The patient should be asked about the nature of the pain, whether it is sharp, dull, or colicky, its relation to bowel action, and the presence of any aggravating or relieving factors. She must be asked if she has noticed any alteration in her bowel habit and questioned about her general state of health. She should also be asked about symptoms likely to be caused by her anaemia, such as angina, dizziness and palpitations.

A history of chronic constipation with abdominal pain and associated bleeding per rectum would suggest diverticulitis. Diarrhoea with blood and mucus, and constitutional symptoms is suggestive of inflammatory bowel disease. Altered bowel habits should alert you to the possibility of a gastrointestinal malignancy: steady weight is reassuring; weight loss with poor appetite suggests a more sinister pathology. Weight gain, lethargy and constipation (which may cause pain in the left iliac fossa) are seen in hypothyroidism.

It would be useful to start with an open-ended question.

Questions

Would you like to tell me about your symptoms as they developed?

How long have you had the pain in your tummy?

Have you had any similar episodes of pain in the past?

What kind of pain is it? — Is it sharp, a dull ache, or does it come in spasms?

Did it come on suddenly or did it build up gradually?

Is it localized to one place or does it travel to anywhere else?

Does anything make it worse?

What happens after a meal?

Does anything relieve it?

Does it get better after a bowel action?

Have you noticed any change in your bowel habits?

Do you have constipation or diarrhoea, or are your bowel movements normal?

Have you ever passed slimy mucus or blood?

Have you ever passed black stools?

How is your appetite?

Is your weight steady?

Have you had any other symptoms?

Has there been any change in your general health?

Has your breathlessness become worse than it was a month ago?

How far can you walk before you become breathless?

Can you climb one flight of stairs without getting breathless?

Do you get any pain in your chest when you walk?

Do you get any dizzy spells?

Is there any family history of bowel problems?

How has it affected your lifestyle?

Do you need any help with your household chores?

Has anyone remarked about your appearance? For example, has anyone said that you look pale?

Have you yourself noticed any change in your complexion?

Mr Thomson is a 50-year-old man who complains about a pain in both his calves on walking about 50 yards. Take a history from him.

History

Although you would need to ask this patient a few more questions about his symptoms, this sounds like *intermittent claudication*, and the most likely cause would be atheromatous peripheral arterial disease. A less likely diagnostic hypothesis, but worth exploring, would be spinal canal stenosis or some form of injury affecting L5/S1 segments. Thromboangiitis obliterans (Buerger's disease) usually affects males between the ages of 20 and 40 years and so is unlikely. The question is about taking a history, rather than simply arriving at a diagnosis, and you should enquire about: risk factors (smoking, blood pressure, diabetes mellitus, hyperlipidaemia, family history, etc.); other manifestations of vascular disease (history of angina or strokes); any history of spinal injury and of any neurological bladder or bowel dysfunction; and drug and social history.

When it comes to taking a history about a complaint such as pain, which takes many forms and has many causes, it is prudent to start with an open-ended question, allowing the patient to describe his complaint freely.

Questions

About the complaint

I understand that you get pain in your legs. Would you like to tell me about it please?

Do you always get the pain on walking or do you sometimes get it when you are resting?

Is it sharp, aching or a squeezing type of pain?

Do you also get it in the thighs or buttocks, or only in the calves?

Do you have to stop walking when you get the pain?

What do you do to relieve the pain? — Do you massage your calves or just sit it out?

How long does it take to wear off before you can walk again?

Does the pain appear again after walking 50 yards or less?

Does anything affect the pain, making it worse or better?

How long have you had this pain?

Has it got any worse with time?

Do you ever get the pain at night in bed? — If so, what do you do to relieve it?

Do you get any other symptoms such as weakness of your muscles, or bladder or bowel trouble?

Have you had any back injuries in the past?

About risk factors and other related problems

Do you smoke?

How many do you smoke a day?

How long have you been smoking?

Do you have any other illnesses?

Have you ever had your blood pressure measured?

Have you ever had your blood cholesterol level measured?

Do you also get chest pain when walking or on any other exertion?

Have you ever had a heart attack?

Have you ever had a sudden weakness on one side?

Is there anybody in the family who had a similar complaint?

Is there any history of high blood pressure, diabetes or strokes in the family?

Are you taking any drugs? (*beta blockers*)

About social history

Does this complaint affect your job?

Does it interfere with your lifestyle?

Do you still do any shopping and other household chores?

Mrs Jones is a 28-year-old housewife and she has postnatal depression. Please take a history from her.

Although the diagnosis of postnatal depression has been mentioned in the question, the candidate must be alert to the fact that this may not be true postpartum depression, but related to one of the following:

- Postpartum blues — many women experience a tearful day soon after delivery but this is transient and they then manage well (*see* case 2.21)
- Substance-related — the patient might feel low for a day or so after delivery as a result of the anaesthetic or sedative given
- Coexisting disorder — she may have had toxaemia or may have an associated disease such as Cushing's syndrome or hypothyroidism

Unlike postnatal 'blues', postnatal depression is characterized by depression and delusions and tends to be persistent, requiring psychotherapy and drugs and, in some cases, electroconvulsive therapy. It develops within 6 weeks of birth; most cases occur within the first 3 weeks; a small proportion of patients develop a depressive illness within the first week of birth. Thoughts of harming the baby or self are a characteristic feature. There is usually a latent period during which the patient appears normal. In its early stages it may be difficult to distinguish from schizophrenia, with similar symptoms and signs, but after 2 to 3 weeks' observation the correct diagnosis should become obvious. With expert treatment the prognosis in most cases is favourable.

History

Questions should be asked about the onset and duration of the depression and about the presence of any associated disorders. If the depression is persistent and demonstrates core symptoms (disturbance of appetite, weight, bowels and sleep; low spirits; and lack of energy), then careful questioning will be needed to distinguish postnatal depression from schizophrenia or preexisting depression. The patient may be feeling trapped in an unhappy marriage and the baby may be either of the unwanted gender or unwanted altogether. She may be uninterested in her surroundings and may even have thoughts of harming the baby. There may be a past or family history of similar episodes. *The Edinburgh Postnatal Depression Scale (EPDS) (see below)* is a useful tool for assessing patients with possible postnatal depression.

Questions

About the complaint

How have you been feeling since the birth of your baby?

Are you feeling low in spirits? — Tell me about it.

Do you cry when you are alone?

How is your appetite?

Have you lost or gained weight?

How are your bowel habits? — Do you have diarrhoea or constipation?

How do you sleep?

Do you find it difficult to go to sleep or do you wake up early?

How long have you been feeling depressed?

How do you feel about the baby?

Are you happy about the baby?

Have you had any similar episodes in the past?

Did you have any problems before the delivery?

Do you have any other complaints or illnesses?

What do you think is wrong with you?

Does anything or anybody have an effect on your thoughts or actions?

Is there anybody in the family who has had a similar experience?

Social history

How does your husband (or partner) feel about your present condition?

Is he supportive and helpful?

Do you feel that the rest of the family is supportive?

How are you coping with the baby?

Do you feel up to doing small household chores?

Edinburgh Postnatal Depression Scale (EPDS)

Name:

Assessor:

Assessment Date:

EPDS Score:

As you have recently had a baby, we would like to know how you are feeling. Please underline the answer which comes closest to how you have felt in the past 7 days — not just how you feel today.

In the past 7 days:

1. **I have been able to laugh and see the funny side of things:**
   As much as I always could
   Not quite so much now
   Definitely not so much now
   Not at all

2. **I have looked forward with enjoyment to things:**
   As much as I ever did
   Rather less than I used to
   Definitely less than I used to
   Hardly at all

3. **I have blamed myself unnecessarily when things went wrong:**
   Yes, most of the time
   Yes, some of the time
   Not very often
   No, never

4. **I have been anxious or worried for no good reason:**
   No, not at all
   Hardly ever
   Yes, sometimes
   Yes, very often

5. **I have felt scared or panicky for no good reason:**
   Yes, quite a lot
   Yes, sometimes
   No, not much
   No, not at all

6. **Things have been getting on top of me:**
   Yes, most of the time I haven't been able to cope at all
   Yes, sometimes I haven't been coping as well as usual
   No, most of the time I have coped quite well
   No, I have been coping as well as ever

7. **I have been so unhappy that I have had difficulty sleeping:**
   Yes, most of the time
   Yes, sometimes
   Not very often
   No, not at all

8. **I have felt sad or miserable:**
   Yes, most of the time
   Yes, quite often
   Not very often
   No, not at all

9. **I have been so unhappy that I have been crying:**
   Yes, most of the time
   Yes, quite often
   Only occasionally
   No, never

10. **The thought of harming myself has occurred to me:**
    Yes, quite often
    Sometimes
    Hardly ever
    Never

Guidelines for raters

Response categories are scored 0,1,2, and 3 according to increased severity of the symptom. Questions 3,5,6,7,8,9,10 are reverse scored (ie, 3,2,1,0). Individual items are totalled to give an overall score. A score of 12+ indicates the likelihood of depression, but not its severity. The EPDS Score is designed to assist, not replace, clinical judgement.

Mrs Moore, a 25-year-old lady, delivered a baby 3 days ago. She is feeling low and tearful. Take a history from her and explain your conclusions to her.

Puerperal mood disorders include maternity 'blues', postnatal depression and postnatal psychosis. This lady is most likely to have maternity 'blues', which characteristically occurs 3–10 days after childbirth. It is fairly common, with a reported incidence between 30% and 80%. Symptoms of maternity 'blues' include depression, labile mood, insomnia, loss of appetite, tiredness, and a feeling of anxiety and irritability. Some patients may present with confusion. Although hormonal imbalances after childbirth, and anxiety or depression in the third trimester of pregnancy may be contributory factors, no definite cause has been identified. It tends to be transient and no active treatment is recommended. Up to 30% of patients may go on to develop postnatal depression. Careful assessment, reassurance, and follow-up of these patients are important.

History

History-taking in this patient would be the same as for postnatal depression (*see* case 2.20). However, you should be ready with questions about her recent emotional state and you are required to explain the diagnosis to the patient and to reassure her. Be gentle and clear in explaining the diagnosis, as it is a particularly stressful time for the patient. Make sure that you have the patient's husband or a family member present during the consultation.

Questions

In the past few days

Have you been able to laugh and see the funny side of things?

Have you looked forward with enjoyment to things generally?

Do you blame yourself unnecessarily when things go wrong?

Do you feel anxious or worried for no good reason?

Have you felt scared or panicky for no good reason?

Do you think that things have been getting on top of you lately?

Do you have difficulty getting to sleep?

Have you felt sad or miserable recently?

Have you felt so unhappy that you have been tearful?

Have you ever thought of harming yourself?

Have you had any difficulty in concentrating?

Do you get support from your family and friends?

Are you finding it difficult to manage with the baby?

How did you feel during the later stage of the preganacy? — Did you feel low at that time?

Did you feel low or depressed before your pregnancy?

Did you have any problems before your periods in the past?

Is there anything else you would like to tell me?

Counselling

Doctor: Mrs Moore, you have been feeling low and tearful. Such a state is very common after pregnancy and is known as maternity 'blues'. This will settle down in a few days' time.

Mrs Moore: What causes maternity 'blues'?

Doctor: The cause for this not entirely known. However, sudden changes in hormone levels after childbirth have been identified as one of the possible reasons. If you had been feeling low during the later stages of the pregnancy, then that can also predispose to maternity 'blues'. As I said before, most women with maternity 'blues' get over it in a few days. No active treatment is necessary. Supportive and understanding family and friends are all that you need. We will, however, need to keep a close eye on things just to make sure that everything goes well because we know that about 30% of patients with maternity 'blues' can develop postnatal depression.

Mrs Moore: Will I develop depression?

Doctor: Most women recover without any long-term effects. So I would not worry too much about that. Here is an information sheet that explains what I have said and also gives you the addresses of the Association of Postnatal Illness and the Meet A Mum Association (MAMA). Both these associations are very supportive and you can contact them if you need any further help.

Mrs Moore: Thank you, doctor.

Doctor: Take care. I will see you again before you go home. Bye for now.

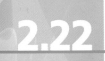

Mr Harkness is a 25-year-old man who has had fever and cough for 2 days. Please take a history from him.

Cough is the commonest clinical presentation of respiratory tract disease. A combination of cough and fever may be either a manifestation of an acute respiratory infection or an acute exacerbation of a chronic respiratory disease.

Acute respiratory diseases

- Upper respiratory tract infection (viral, bacterial)
  — Acute laryngitis
  — Acute tracheitis
  — Acute tracheobronchitis
- Lower respiratory tract infection (e.g. pneumonia)
  — Infective (bacterial, viral, atypical organisms, TB)
  — Chemical (aspiration pneumonia)
  — Post-radiation pneumonitis
  — Allergic mechanisms — simple and prolonged pulmonary eosinophilia, asthmatic bronchopulmonary eosinophilia
- Bronchial asthma (acute attack)

Acute exacerbations of chronic lung diseases

- Chronic obstructive airways disease
- Bronchiectasis
- Asthma
- Sarcoidosis
- Pulmonary fibrosis

Other causes of cough

- Carcinoma of the lung

■ Drugs (ACE inhibitors, beta-blockers)
■ Psychological

History

When eliciting a history from a patient with respiratory symptoms it is important to know about their previous health. A detailed assessment of the presenting symptoms and associated symptoms will usually provide clues to the diagnosis. When questioning about the cough the patient should be asked about its onset, duration, time of occurrence, any change in frequency or severity, and about any associated features (e.g. the harsh, barking quality of laryngitis or the bovine cough of vocal cord paralysis).

Expectoration is an important feature of most respiratory diseases. Detailed information should be obtained about the quantity and colour (mucoid in chronic bronchitis; yellow/green in infection; rusty in pneumonia; pink and frothy in acute pulmonary oedema; black in smokers; and blood stained in cancer, TB, and acute bronchitis).

Your history should also include an enquiry about other symptoms such as breathlessness, chest pain, wheeze, and haemoptysis, and questions about past medical history and family history.

Questions

Would you tell me all you can about your complaints, please?

Were you fit and well before these last 2 days?

Did the cough start suddenly or gradually?

Is it constant or does it occur at a particular time of the day?

What brings it on?

Have you noticed any strange quality to your cough?

Are you coughing up any phlegm?

If yes — How much do you cough up, an eggcupful, or a teacupful?

What colour is the phlegm?

Have you noticed any blood in the phlegm?

Have you had any drenching sweats with feeling hot and cold, or with rigors?

Do you have any chest pains?

Have you been breathless or wheezy?

Have you lost any weight?

Have you ever had TB, pneumonia or asthma?

Have you been in contact with anybody with TB recently?

Rarely, these symptoms may be caused by unusual viral infections such as HIV, the virus that causes AIDS. Are you aware of any risk factors that you may have for HIV infection, such as haemophilia, blood transfusions, intravenous drug use, or unprotected sex?

Do you have any other medical problems?

Are you on any medication?

Do you smoke?

Have you ever smoked?

Have you been abroad recently and stayed in a hotel with air-conditioned rooms?

Does anyone in your family have any chest diseases?

Mrs Girdwood, a 22-year-old lady, complains of breathlessness and wheezing. You suspect she has asthma. Take a history to confirm the diagnosis.

Although a possible diagnosis of asthma has been suggested in the question, you should not overlook other conditions with these presenting symptoms, even though some of these are very unlikely possibilities:

- Left heart failure
- Chronic obstructive airways disease
- Tumour causing airway obstruction
- Functional/psychogenic
- Rare causes — carcinoid syndrome, infiltrative airways disease (amyloid, sarcoid), pulmonary embolism

History

In a young patient the most likely diagnosis would be *bronchial asthma*. A history suggestive of underlying asthma includes: wheezing (the cardinal symptom of asthma); cough (this may be the only symptom in adults); and worsening of symptoms at night or in the early hours of the morning ('morning dip' — an exaggeration of the natural circadian rhythm). There may be a history of childhood asthma, hay fever, or eczema (i.e. atopy), and a family history of asthma.

Questions

Would you like to describe your complaints to me?

When did you first start having breathlessness and wheezing?

Do you have a cough?

If yes — Is the cough constant or do you cough just when you have a wheezy episode?

Are your symptoms worse in the middle of the night or the early hours of the morning?

Do you get breathless and wheezy when you are walking or exercising?

Does cold air or a smoky environment affect your symptoms?

Did you have asthma, hay fever, or eczema as a child?

Does anybody in your family suffer from asthma?

Are you taking any medication? (*aspirin and beta-blockers can aggravate asthma*)

Do you have any other medical problems?

Ross is a 3-year-old boy. His mother complains that he is not growing well, is drinking a lot of water, and is feeling ill. Please take a history from her.

The history of failure to thrive and polydipsia bring to mind a well-defined group of conditions (*diabetes mellitus, diabetes insipidus, hypercalcaemia* from any cause, and *psychogenic polydipsia*), but you must not lose sight of the fact that the child may have some other systemic disorder, such as an endocrine problem, malabsorption, infection, or a chronic system failure. Diabetes insipidus in a child may be caused by a craniopharyngioma or may be part of the Hand–Schüller–Christian disease (characterized by lytic skull lesions, exophthalmos and diabetes insipidus).

History

Ross may just be a constitutionally small child, or slow to grow, but the mother says that he is unwell and is drinking excessive amounts of water. Even though there is a bewildering number of conditions that may affect a child's growth and well-being, the most likely diagnosis is either diabetes mellitus or diabetes insipidus. Find out first if Ross is really not growing well, by reference to a height and weight against age chart, and once this has been established, ask further questions to try and identify the underlying problem.

Questions

Do you think Ross is small for his age and sex?

Have you kept a record of his weight and height and, if so, may I please have a look at it?

Would you like to tell me what you mean when you say that Ross is unwell?

How long has he been unwell?

How long have you noticed that he is not growing?

Has he been slow in gaining weight or has he lost weight?

Tell me about his drinking habits.

Do you know how much he drinks in a day?

How long has he been drinking excessively?

How much water does he pass in a day?

Does he wet his bed at night?

How is his appetite?

Does he eat more or less than you expect him to eat?

Have you noticed anything unusual or any lumps on his head or body?

How was your health during and after the pregnancy?

What was his birth weight?

Does Ross have any other illnesses, such as chest infections, thyroid disease or asthma?

Is he on any medication?

Is there anybody in the family with diabetes?

Have you got any other children?

If yes — Have they had similar problems in the past?

How does Ross compare with them at a comparable age?

Mr White complains of pains in his joints. Take a history in order to arrive at a differential diagnosis.

Although his age is not stated, this patient is most probably an adult, so any childhood causes of joint pain can be excluded from the differential diagnosis. The age of the patient and the joints involved can be useful indicators of the possible diagnosis. From the brief history given it seems unlikely that this is a monarticular joint disorder.

From his age group you will be able to narrow down the number of possible joint disorders he may have:

- Young male
  — Ankylosing spondylitis
  — Adult Still's disease
  — Reiter's syndrome
- Middle-aged male
  — Rheumatoid arthritis (RA)
  — Gout
- Older male
  — Rheumatoid arthritis
  — Osteoarthrosis (OA)
  — Gout

Other causes of joint pains include:

- Psoriatic arthropathy
- Septic arthritis (usually monarticular)
- Hypertrophic pulmonary osteoarthropathy (HPOA)
- Ulcerative colitis/Crohn's disease
- Sickle cell disease

History

Age, sex (RA is more common in women; Reiter's syndrome is more common in men), and race (e.g. sickle cell disease in Afro-Caribbeans) are obvious clues to the underlying cause. It is not particularly helpful to ask questions about the *type* of pain because all joint pains feel much the same to most patients. It is important to elucidate the joints involved (fingers in RA and psoriasis; hands, hips, and knees in OA; wrists in HPOA; toes in gout; sacroiliac joints in ankylosing spondylitis) and the duration of symptoms (long in RA; short in gout).

Joint pain in acute gout comes on suddenly and is severe; in RA, OA, and psoriasis it gets gradually worse. Inflammatory joint pains are relieved by activity; mechanical problems are made worse by activity and are relieved by rest. Inflammatory joint pain is worse in the morning and improves during the day and morning stiffness is characteristic of inflammatory arthropathy. A lesion in the cervical or lumbar spine can give pain in the distribution of the affected nerve roots.

A history of associated symptoms such as joint swelling, increasing immobility, general lethargy, skin rash, red eyes, fever, shortness of breath, nodules, or bowel disturbance may be useful. Any family history of joint problems (OA, ankylosing spondylitis, gout) and the social history (occupation, for example, can be a factor in OA) should be explored. Ask about any previous treatment (e.g. NSAIDs, gold, methotrexate, indometacin).

Questions

Would you please tell me something about your joint pains?

Which joints are painful?

How long have the joints been painful?

Did the pain come on suddenly or did it gradually get worse?

How often are the joints painful and how long does the pain last?

Is the pain worse at rest or when you move about?

Is the pain worse in the morning?

Does the pain get less severe when you limber up?

Does the pain move anywhere else?

Do you have any morning stiffness?
Do you have any other symptoms?
Have you had any skin rashes or lumps?
Have you had any problems with your eyes?
Have you been short of breath?
Have you had any problems with your bowels lately?
Have you had any other medical problems in the past?
Are you on any medication?
Does anyone in your family have joint problems?
How old are you?
What is your occupation?
Do the joint pains affect your work or your social activities?
How does the family cope with your disability?

Mr Martins is a 63-year-old man referred to the Memory Clinic. Would you perform a Mini Mental State (MMS) examination?

If you are asked to do this, then it is likely that the patient is confused (i.e. has a cognitive defect of some kind) or, if he is a healthy volunteer, he will have been suitably tutored to demonstrate a defect. In clinical practice, an *acute confusional state* may be caused by infection, myocardial infarction, electrolyte imbalance, hypercalcaemia, alcohol or drug intoxication or there may be a chronic condition such as *Alzheimer's disease* or *multi-infarct dementia* (recurrent cerebrovascular events causing a step-wise deterioration in mental capacity). It is well to remember these causes as you may be asked about them.

History

Generally, in an exam situation, the *abbreviated MMS examination* should be used and you should ask the patient:

1. His age
2. The time of day
3. To recall an address at the end of the test (Give him an address early on and ask him to repeat this straight away to ensure that he has heard it correctly.)
4. The year
5. The name of the place where you are
6. To recognize two people (e.g. doctor and nurse — choose two people in the immediate surroundings whose occupation is easily recognizable)
7. His date of birth (the date and month are sufficient)
8. The dates of the First World War
9. The name of the present monarch or prime minister
10. To count backwards from 20 to 1

Each correct answer scores 1 mark and cognitive function is graded as severely impaired (0–3 marks), moderately impaired (4–7 marks), or normal (8–10 marks). This is an initial screening tool and does not provide enough information to differentiate between acute and chronic confusional states. Further investigation would be needed to establish a cause.

Remember that patients who have a speech problem may have normal memory and cognitive function but still perform badly on these tests. Other factors, such as drowsiness, alcohol, drugs, or surrounding noise can also affect performance.

Questions

May I ask you how old you are?

Without looking at a watch, can you tell to the nearest hour what time it is now?

I am going to give you an address. After I have finished saying it to you, I want you to repeat it. Then try and remember what the address is because I'll ask you again in a few minutes. The address is '24 West Register Street'. Would you repeat it please … good!

Can you tell me what year it is?

Could you tell me the name of this place where we are now?

Can you recognize who these two people are? *(point out two easily recognizable people, e.g. a doctor and a nurse)*

What is your date of birth?

What are the dates of the First World War?

Who is the prime minister now?

Could you count backwards from 20 to 1?

What is the address that I asked you to repeat a few minutes ago?

2.27

Mr Watson, a 70-year-old man, had an episode of weakness of his right hand that lasted for half an hour and recovery was complete. Assess the risk factors for a transient ischaemic attack (TIA) in this patient and explain the diagnosis and management to him.

This history does sound very suggestive of a TIA, causing weakness of short duration (i.e. resolving in less than 24 hours).

History

The *risk factors* that need to be assessed (for diagnosis and for secondary prevention) in the history include:

- Age of the patient (usually elderly, occasionally middle-aged)
- Hypertension
- Smoking (cigarettes carry a higher risk than pipe smoking)
- Obesity
- Hyperlipidaemia
- Past history of a TIA or stroke
- Family history of TIAs, strokes, heart disease, high cholesterol
- Diabetes mellitus
- Atrial fibrillation
- Recent myocardial infarction
- Cardiac source of embolus
- Carotid artery stenosis
- High plasma viscosity (polycythaemia rubra vera, myeloma, hypertriglyceridaemia, Waldenström's macroglobulinaemia)

Questions

Have you had these episodes before?

If yes — How many, and how long did each episode last?

Have you had any episodes affecting other parts of your body?

Have you had any other symptoms?

Have you ever had any palpitations or chest pain?

Do you ever get dizzy?

Do you keep a record of your weight?

What is your most recent weight?

Do you smoke?

If yes — What do you smoke?

How many cigarettes do you smoke a day, or how much tobacco a week?

How long have you been smoking?

Have you had high blood pressure?

Are you a diabetic?

Have you ever been told that you had a raised cholesterol level?

Have you ever had any problems with your heart? — If so, what?

Do you have any other medical problems?

Has anyone in your family had TIAs, strokes, heart disease, or high cholesterol? (you may have to explain what you mean by a TIA)

Counselling

Doctor: Mr Watson, thank you for your patience. You have a condition called 'transient ischaemic attack', in which you feel a weakness of some part of the body, as you felt in your right hand. It is temporary but may last for up to 24 hours. It happens when a blood vessel to a part of the brain becomes temporarily blocked but opens up again.

Mr Watson: Is it likely to happen again and am I likely to have a stroke?

Doctor: I'm afraid the answer to both these questions is yes, though you may never have any further trouble again. However, you can do a lot to reduce the chances of such an event. I would like to do a few tests before we can consider any treatment. I will have to take a few blood samples to check your full blood count, blood sugar, blood lipids, and do a clotting screen. I will also arrange a CT scan of the brain. Whatever the results of these tests, I'm afraid you will have to give up smoking for good and adopt a more healthy lifestyle by reducing the fat content of your diet and increasing your physical activity.

I will arrange these investigations and refer you to our physiotherapist for an exercise programme. I will discuss some of these things again with you. Is there anything that I have not mentioned or that you would like to bring up?

Mr Watson: No, doctor, not at the moment. Thank you.

Mr Holmes, a 50-year-old accountant, has been having pain in his chest on walking over the past 2 months. Please take a history from him.

History

Although the wording here suggests that this patient has angina of effort — and questions should be directed primarily at elucidating that — other diagnostic possibilities, such as oesophageal or musculoskeletal pain, should be borne in mind. Explore the characteristics of the pain first to establish if it is of cardiac origin. If the patient's answers point to one of the other possible causes then you will need to redirect your questions.

The age of the patient and his stressful occupation are helpful pointers here to ischaemic heart disease and your enquiry should be extended to assess other risk factors, such as previous episodes of angina, smoking, and personal or family history of hypertension or hypercholesterolaemia. It is particularly important to cover all the possible risk factors because you are being asked to take a history and not simply to make a diagnosis.

Questions

About the pain

Tell me exactly what happens when you walk?

Would you describe this pain for me please?

Is it sharp, dull, gripping, burning, or a pressing sensation?

Can you show me exactly where you feel it in your chest?

Does it spread anywhere else? — If so, where to?

How long does it last?

Do you always get the pain on walking or do you get it when you are resting as well?

Does anything else bring it on? — For example, do you get it when you are angry, excited or if someone makes an unpleasant phone call?

Does eating any particular food bring it on?

Do you get it after a meal or on bending or turning?

How long do you have to walk before you get the pain? — How about when you are walking up an incline or going upstairs?

Does the pain always ease up when you rest?

Does it start again when you start walking again?

Does anything else ease the pain?

When did you first start having the pain?

Has it been getting any worse? — For example, is it more easily induced or more severe now?

Do you get any other symptoms when you get this pain?

Have you had any similar episodes in the past?

About the risk factors

Tell me about your smoking habits, whether you smoke now, or used to smoke.

How much do you smoke? — I mean, how many cigarettes a day or how much tobacco a week?

Have you had a medical examination recently for any reason?

Have you ever had your blood pressure measured?

Has anyone measured your blood cholesterol level?

Do you experience stress in your job?

Is your pain related to times when your clients overload you with their tax returns?

Is there any family history of heart trouble or high blood pressure?

Mrs Maitland is a 30-year-old lady with a 6-month history of constipation, with bouts of diarrhoea and abdominal pain. Please take a history from her.

Constipation, diarrhoea, and abdominal pains are the classic symptoms of the *irritable bowel syndrome*. This is the diagnosis you will be expected to establish but along the way there are many problems — each symptom needs to be explored fully and each one has its own set of differential diagnoses. The main differential diagnosis of the irritable bowel syndrome comprises:

- Malabsorption
- Peptic ulcer disease
- Gall bladder disease
- Rectosigmoid tumour
- Chronic pelvic inflammatory disease
- Hyperthyroidism

An understanding of this syndrome is essential for planning your questions and arriving at a diagnosis. There is a significant psychogenic component in most patients with the irritable bowel syndrome and it may seem difficult to pin down the exact nature of each symptom on closer questioning.

Constipation is the most persistent of the three complaints in this condition and, regardless of the age at presentation, it dates back to the late teens in most patients. These patients tend to be overoccupied with their bowels and may complain of having periods when they have loose motions as well as their usual experience of hard and infrequent stools. Some patients pass 'pencil' stools, suggestive of high tone in the anal sphincter, which is easily distinguishable from the constipation of hypothyroidism and rectal malignancy.

Over the years most patients with the irritable bowel syndrome complain of *abdominal pains and cramps*. The pains are characteristically poorly localized along the course of the colon, although some patients point towards the right upper quadrant. The pain may last for anything between a few minutes and many hours, may be brought on by certain foods (such as strong spicy dishes, fruits, and vegetables), and is often relieved by the passage of gas. The pain gradually assumes more importance than the disordered bowel function and, depending on the principal location, may be confused with that of gall bladder disease, peptic ulcer disease, or ileocaecal or sigmoid colon pathology.

Diarrhoea may be initiated by an episode of gastroenteritis or food poisoning. There may be only one or two loose motions in the day or an explosive series of ten or more stools after breakfast in response to the gastrocolic reflex. It is not unusual for patients to blame alcohol or coffee for inducing the diarrhoea. Often there is no more diarrhoea after the initial bout in the mornings, and there is seldom any during the night (when it would be inconvenient). Some patients have periods of constipation alternating with periods of diarrhoea. Sometimes patients pass mucus which they may confuse with worms or pus. In such cases, particularly when diarrhoea is the predominant symptom, villous adenoma or rectosigmoid polyp will have to be excluded.

History

Starting with the three cardinal symptoms of constipation, abdominal pain and diarrhoea, it should be possible to establish the diagnosis of the irritable bowel syndrome without much difficulty. However, candidates should keep in mind the all the other conditions that cause these symptoms and these may need to be explored, depending on the answers given by the patient.

Tactful questioning often reveals emotional stress which is fundamental to the irritable bowel syndrome. The patients may have had strict toilet-training during their early childhood; they may be highly strung and prone to diarrhoea during stress; and there may be other social, emotional, sexual or financial problems.

Questions

About the symptoms

Please could you give me some details about your complaints, starting with how and when they developed?

How long have you had the constipation?

When you are constipated how long do you go without opening your bowels?

Do you experience any difficulty in passing a motion?

What do your stools look like?

Do you pass any mucus or blood?

How long do the bouts of diarrhoea and constipation last?

Are you mostly constipated, regular, or does the diarrhoea predominate?

Is the diarrhoea more frequent at any particular times?

Do you ever get diarrhoea during the night?

Does anything make the diarrhoea or abdominal pain worse?

Does anything relieve the pain?

Where exactly do you get the abdominal pain?

What does the pain feel like? — Is it a dull ache, a sharp pain or like a cramp?

You said that you don't get any diarrhoea after the morning bout. — Is that true for the weekends as well as for weekdays?

Psychosocial history

Are there any times when you have none of the three complaints you mentioned? — If so, is there anything special about those times?

Are there any times when the complaints are at their worst?

Do you remember anything about your bowel habits in your childhood?

Do you have any memory of your toilet-training?

Do you have any hobbies? If so, does the diarrhoea ever interfere with them?

Do you ever get diarrhoea when you are stressed for any reason?

Do you have any symptoms when you are on holiday with your family?

Can you think of anything that might be causing stress at home?

Did you have any particularly difficult or, on the other hand, trouble-free periods in your life? — For example, how did your bowels behave when you left home, at the time of your marriage, or when you had your children?

Mrs Leslie, a 32-year-old lady, has had bleeding per vaginam recently and a pain in her abdomen for the last 3 hours. Please take a history from her.

In a lady of childbearing age with these symptoms, one has first to consider ectopic pregnancy and miscarriage. If the abdominal pain is a recurrent problem there is a wider differential diagnosis:

- Ectopic pregnancy
- Miscarriage
- Rupture of an ovarian cyst
- Secondary dysmenorrhoea — adenomyosis, endometriosis, chronic sepsis
- Fibroids (torsion of a pedunculated fibroid)
- Cervical cancer

History

A detailed menstrual history is crucial to explore the possibility of a pregnancy. Acute *ectopic pregnancy* presents with shock or syncope but subacute cases often present with the classic triad of abdominal pain, vaginal bleeding and amenorrhoea, as in the scenario given here. In ectopic pregnancy there is usually an 8-week history of amenorrhoea, although an ectopic can present before a period is missed. Abdominal pain usually precedes the vaginal bleeding (which may be dark, 'like prune juice', or fresh). The pain may be referred to the shoulder, and felt on defaecation or when passing water. Enquiry should also be made about the presence of any risk factors such as a history of previous ectopic pregnancy, pelvic inflammatory disease, smoking, douching, or the use of an intrauterine device.

In *miscarriage* there may be a history of missed periods or the patient may feel that she is having a period but that the pain and bleeding are worse than during a normal period. She may report passing bits of tissue mixed with the blood.

Secondary dysmenorrhoea is unlikely in a 32-year-old lady and the pain tends to be constant throughout the period. There is usually a history of pain with previous menstrual cycles as well. Advanced carcinoma of the cervix can present with bleeding and abdominal pain but this is rare these days with the availability of cervical smear screening. A history of postcoital bleeding is suggestive of cervical trauma, polyps, vaginitis, or cancer of the cervix. Questions should be asked about systemic symptoms such as fever, weight loss, and loss of appetite.

Questions

When did you last have a period?

If she has missed any periods:
Do you know of any reason why your periods have stopped?'
Is there any chance that you may be pregnant?
(*The patient may admit to the likelihood of conception; otherwise you may have to ask a few more questions.*)
Have you had unprotected sex recently?
Have you missed taking the pill recently?
Did the tummy pain come before the bleeding?
Is the bleeding dark or fresh?
Do you have any pain anywhere else?
Do you have any shoulder-tip pain?
Do you have any pain on opening your bowels or when passing water?
Is this bleeding like your periods or is it more severe than your usual periods?
Have you passed any clots?
Have you noticed any bits of tissue other than clots?
Have you had an ectopic pregnancy in the past? — If so, are your symptoms now the same as they were then?
Have you ever used an intrauterine device?

Have you ever had any infection either of the womb or the tubes?

Are you a smoker or an ex-smoker?

If she has not missed any periods you still have to ask many of the above questions and then follow up with some of the following questions:

Have your periods been regular or irregular?

How many days does the flow last?

How many pads do you normally use?

Have you passed any clots before?

Do you always have pains with your periods? — If so, does the pain last throughout the period?

Have you noticed any bleeding in-between your periods?

Have you noticed any spotting or bleeding after sex?

Have you had any fever, drenching sweats, or rigors recently?

How is your appetite?

Have you lost any weight?

Do you have any other medical problems?

Are you on any medication?

Mrs Hunt is a 36-year-old lady with anxiety. Please take a history from her.

This opening statement is somewhat vague and does not state if she has volunteered that she is anxious, or whether she is in a constant state of anxiety or is experiencing acute attacks of anxiety or panic (with apprehension, sweating, dryness of the mouth, trembling, discomfort in the chest, etc.). The vagueness is probably deliberate and designed to test your history-taking skills. You have not been told, for example, whether her anxiety is a secondary manifestation of a medical or surgical condition, or if it is the primary or predominant symptom.

Before embarking on taking a history of her presenting complaints, you should remind yourself of two important facts about anxiety. First, anxiety may be a normal and appropriate response and it can enhance concentration and effort. Second, anxiety may be a prominent manifestation of some medical disorders (acute toxic confusion, thyrotoxicosis, phaeochromocytoma, and hypoglycaemia), and it can be part, though not the main component, of almost any psychiatric disorder (e.g. depressive states, schizophrenia, presenile and senile dementia, drugs or alcohol abuse, post-concussion syndromes). In summary, anxiety disorders may be:

- An exaggerated psychosomatic response to stressful situations
- Associated with any medical or surgical condition
- The chief component of a clinical syndrome
- A prominent feature of a psychiatric condition

History

The purpose of taking a history from this patient is first to confirm that she does have anxiety, and then to try and determine the cause of it. Anxiety can have multisystem manifestations and you should find out if the patient has any musculoskeletal symptoms (tremor, general aches and pains, headaches, or pain in the back or neck); cardiovascular symptoms (palpitations, precordial pain); respiratory symptoms (breathlessness, sighing, poor effort tolerance); gastrointestinal symptoms (dry mouth, epigastric tremulousness or 'butterflies', dyspepsia, abdominal pain, constipation, or diarrhoea); or sudomotor symptoms (increased sweating).

Ask the patient about any predisposing or precipitating factors and if her sleep and work are disturbed. Find out how she perceives her illness and if there is any family history of anxiety. Any symptoms suggestive of medical or psychiatric disease should be explored. If the anxiety is intermittent and arises in particular circumstances, the patient has a *phobic anxiety disorder*. In this condition patients avoid situations that provoke anxiety, such as crowds or open spaces (agoraphobia), heights (acrophobia) or spiders (arachnophobia).

Questions

Please give me some idea about your symptoms and the circumstances in which they arise.

When were you last fully well and how did your symptoms start?

Do you get any headaches or any other aches and pains in the body?

Are you ever aware of symptoms such as tremulousness, palpitations, dry mouth, or increased sweating?

What circumstances bring these symptoms on and what brought them on when they first appeared?

Is there anything you can do to relieve or stop these symptoms?

Do you have any reason to be apprehensive about the state of your health?

What do you think is wrong with you?

Do you have any fears or worries?

Do you get any panic attacks, and if so, what brings them on?

Do you get depressed?

How well do you sleep?

Have you had any other illnesses?

Is there any family history of any nervous illness?

Do these symptoms stop you from working normally?

Do you take any medicines?

How much do you drink a week?

How do you get on with other people?

Is there anything you want to tell me that we have not discussed?

Mrs Jenkins, a 20-year-old fitness instructor, is referred with a murmur heard over her precordium. Please ask her some relevant questions.

This is an interesting scenario in which the examiner has cleverly provided three clues that may help you to narrow down the differential diagnosis. Firstly, we are not told why the patient presented to the doctor who discovered the murmur, but the implication is that she is asymptomatic and that it is the murmur which has concerned the referring doctor. She is young and fit and one can therefore discount the 'innocent' murmurs caused by an increased flow through the outflow tract valves in conditions such as anaemia, thyrotoxicosis, and pregnancy, or found in association with skeletal abnormalities such as kyphoscoliosis and funnel chest. She is too young to have atherosclerosis (aortic sclerosis), ischaemic heart disease (papillary muscle dysfunction), or atrial myxoma, and too well to have infective endocarditis or a collagen disease.

Secondly, we can safely assume that there is no history of rheumatic fever as the referring doctor would have discovered that. The doctor would also have asked her if anyone had heard a murmur either at birth or afterwards. She must have had a medical examination before she got her job as a fitness instructor and it is unlikely that she would have been passed fit if there was a significant auscultatory finding.

Thirdly, young athletic subjects are occasionally found to have a systolic murmur which turns out to be a sign of hypertrophic obstructive cardiomyopathy.

A systolic murmur over the pulmonary area (mild pulmonary stenosis, atrial septal defect) or over the mitral area (mitral valve prolapse) may not have been loud enough in the past to have caused any alarm at earlier examinations.

The main differential diagnosis is therefore:

- Hypertrophic cardiomyopathy
- Pulmonary stenosis
- Mitral valve prolapse
- Atrial septal defect

History

The essence of history-taking here is to test these assumptions and rule out the conditions you think are unlikely to be the cause of this lady's murmur. You should find out if and when she has been examined in the past and what she was told, and if she has developed any symptoms such as dyspnoea, chest pain, palpitations or syncope.

Questions

Did you have a medical examination before starting your present job and were you told anything about a murmur then?

Have you ever had a medical examination in the past and been told anything?

Has anyone previously heard a murmur over your heart?

Did you have rheumatic fever or growing pains as a child?

Have you ever been investigated for a heart murmur?

(*If she answers 'yes' to any of these questions, get further details before assessing her symptoms.*)

Do you have any chest pains or discomfort?

If yes — How long have you been getting the pain?

Where is the pain when you have it?

What kind of pain is it? — Is it a constricting, sharp, squeezing, crushing or pressing sort of a pain?

Does it spread anywhere?

How long does it last?

What brings it on?

Does anything that you do ease the pain?

Have you been short of breath recently?

If yes — How long for?

Does it come on suddenly or gradually?

Does anything make it worse?

Have you ever woken from sleep trying to catch your breath? (*paroxysmal nocturnal dyspnoea*)

Can you sleep lying flat? — How many pillows do you use?

Have you increased the number of pillows recently? (*orthopnoea*)

Have you ever felt dizzy or have you ever passed out?

If yes — Tell me what actually happened.

Have you ever felt your heart thumping? (*palpitations*)

If yes — Does it start suddenly or gradually?

Does the sensation pass away gradually or suddenly?

Can you tap it out on the table as you feel it?

Can you get on with your job as a fitness instructor comfortably?

Have you ever been pregnant?

If yes — Did you have any symptoms such as undue breathlessness during the pregnancy?

Did the doctor who examined you then mention a heart murmur?

Does anyone in your family have any heart problems?

Amanda is a 6-year-old girl and she has had an earache in her left ear for 2 days. Ask her and her anxious mother some questions.

The main issue here is to determine the cause of the earache so that it can be successfully treated. When considering the possible causes keep in mind the three principal disease processes — traumatic, inflammatory and neoplastic — and the anatomy of the ear. In a young person you should think of:

- *Pinna* — haematoma, laceration, herpes zoster oticus
- *External auditory meatus* — otitis externa, trauma, infection from swimming, impetigo, erysipelas, boils, dermatoses
- *Middle ear* — traumatic perforation of the drum (e.g. bomb blast), foreign body, instrumentation, myringitis bullosa (Coxsackie B virus), acute suppurative otitis media, acute mastoiditis, fracture of the temporal bone
- *Referred otalgia* — pain referred from disease in the naso-, oro- or hypopharynx, posterior molars, or the temporomandibular joint

History

Earache is distressing, not only for the child who is suffering, but also for the parents, who tend to be very anxious about the possibility that there might be something seriously wrong inside the child's head. During the initial pleasantries, while you briefly consider the possible causes of the earache and the questions you need to ask, you should reassure both the child and the mother.

Questions

To the child

Come and sit here next to me, Amanda. I am going to have a look into your ear and I am sure that we will be able to make it better, but first I must ask you a few questions. Show me exactly where it hurts.

How did it start? — Did you hurt yourself or did you put anything in your ear?

Have you been swimming and did any water get into your ear?

Is it an ache or a sharp pain?

Is it there all the time or does it come and go?

Does it feel sore to touch, and if so, where?

Does the pain go anywhere else?

Do you have any pains anywhere else?

Have you had a sore throat or a toothache?

Do you get the pain when you chew or swallow?

Does anything come out of the ear? — If so, what does it look like?

To the mother

Does Amanda get earaches very often?

Was she out of sorts or did she have any aches and pains before it started?

Did you see anything on the pillow that may have oozed out of the ear?

Does Amanda have any skin conditions?

A mother brings in her 7-year-old son, Michael, with a runny nose. Ask her some questions.

A runny nose, or *rhinorrhoea*, is a common complaint in early childhood, though not one that a mother would rush to a doctor for unless there was a special reason, such as persistent, foul-smelling or bloodstained nasal discharge. It is helpful, therefore, to classify the causes of rhinorrhoea according to the *type of discharge*:

- Watery — early viral infection (common cold), allergy, vasomotor rhinitis
- Mucus and mucopus — acute and chronic rhinitis with or without sinusitis
- CSF — fractured skull
- Foul-smelling (unilateral) — foreign body (may have learning disability)
- Bloodstained — trauma, chronic infection, polyps

History

You have been asked here to question just the mother. There may be a special reason why she has become anxious about her son's runny nose — it may have persisted beyond a few days or the nature of the discharge may be worrying her. You should bear this in mind while considering what questions you are going to ask. As with most conditions of the ear, nose and throat, the diagnosis will be established on inspection, but a few well-chosen questions can make a significant contribution.

Questions

How long has Michael had a runny nose?

What is the discharge like? — Is there any blood or pus or is it just watery?

Is the discharge smelly?

Does the discharge come from one or both nostrils?

Does he get any bouts of sneezing? (*vasomotor rhinitis*)

Is there any seasonal effect on his runny nose? (*hay fever*)

Does he have any fever with his runny nose?

Has he had any injury?

Has he complained of headache or pain in his face? (*sinusitis*)

Are you aware of him having put anything up his nose?

A mother has brought in her 8-year-old son, Peter, with a sore throat. Ask them some questions.

A sore throat is one of the commonest complaints encountered by general practitioners in the UK. The vast majority are caused by a self-limiting viral infection. Improving nutritional, social, and health standards and the widespread use of antibiotics have reduced the incidence of pharyngeal infections and tonsillitis, but there are still around 100 000 tonsillectomies carried out every year in this country.

Acute and chronic pharyngitis and *tonsillitis* account for most cases of a sore throat in young children:

- Viral pharyngitis — influenza viruses, parainfluenza viruses, rhinoviruses, adenoviruses, Coxsackieviruses, and herpesviruses
- Tonsillitis — β-haemolytic streptococci, pneumococci, *Haemophilus influenzae,* and gonococcus
- Infectious mononucleosis — Epstein–Barr virus
- Other infections — *Candida,* toxoplasmosis and tuberculosis

There are a small number of *non-infectious causes* of sore throat:

- Postnasal drip — allergic rhinitis, vasomotor rhinitis, and sinusitis
- Chemical irritation — tobacco (passive smoking), fumes, and dust
- Foreign body — e.g. fish bones

History

Acute pharyngitis is a brief, self-limiting condition and causes soreness of the throat and a cough which is sometimes productive of sputum. Patients with chronic pharyngitis complain of a dull and persistent sore throat, which is often worse in the mornings. Acute follicular tonsillitis is a common condition in childhood and causes sore throat, painful swallowing, pyrexia (sometimes with rigors and delirium), systemic upset, and otalgia; some patients also have halitosis (bad breath).

Questions

To Peter

How are you feeling today, Peter? — Tell me about your problem.

How is your throat now?

Do you feel any soreness in your throat?

Tell me how it all started.

How long have you had it for?

Do you have any difficulty swallowing?

Do you have a pain anywhere else?

Do you have a cough and if so, do you bring up anything?

Have you had something similar in the past?

To the mother

Would you like to add anything to what Peter has told me?

Does anyone else in the family get sore throats?

How often does he get sore throats?

Does he get a temperature with his sore throat?

Does Peter get any other symptoms with it?

Does his breath smell when he has a sore throat?

Does he ever get bouts of coughing at night? (*postnasal drip*)

Susan, a 14-year-old schoolgirl, comes from school with a painful, red eye. Please take a history from her.

During their surgical attachments most students will have some exposure to ophthalmology clinics and receive some teaching on diseases of the eye. Although you will probably not be expected to make an accurate diagnosis from the history alone, the examiners will be assessing your knowledge of the conditions which cause a red eye, and they will be interested in how you pursue the various diagnostic possibilities. Before embarking on your history you should try and recall the various *causes of a red eye*:

- *Conjunctival suffusion* — conjunctivitis (allergic, viral, bacterial, parasitic), trauma, foreign body
- *Corneo-scleral injection* — iritis, corneal abrasion, trauma, foreign body, acute glaucoma (unlikely at this age)

  Associated symptoms:

- Pain
- Watering
- Some disturbance of vision
- Headache
- Discharge — watery, mucopurulent

History

Although you should bear these conditions in mind when planning your questions, you are in fact given an important pointer in the question; namely that she is coming directly to her doctor from school. It would be reasonable to assume that she went to school with a normal eye and that something happened at school to cause the pain and redness in her eye. This raises the possibility of trauma or of a foreign body, or toxic fluid may have been splashed into the eye during a science lesson. The presence of pain suggests that she may have some corneal abrasion. Although a possible incident at school is worth enquiring about, you should also consider the possibility that she might have had very mild conjunctivitis in the morning which has become much worse as the day has progressed.

Questions

Have you had a red eye for some time or did it happen today?

If today:

Tell me what happened.

Did you have any itching or discomfort in the eye when you woke up this morning?

Do you have a sharp pain or does it feel like some grit in your eye?

Does it hurt to open your eye?

Have you hurt your eye or did anything get splashed into your eye?

If the eye has been red for some time:

Can you tell me how long it has been red?

Did it start suddenly or gradually?

Has it been getting worse?

Have you had any trouble in the other eye?

Have you had any discharge? — If so, what kind?

Have you had any similar trouble before?

You are the SHO in the Casualty Unit where you see a 70-year-old man complaining of pain in his abdomen. He is known to have a pulsatile abdominal aneurysm that was diagnosed by ultrasound last year. He is being followed up by a surgical team but because of this sudden pain he has come in as an emergency. Please take a history from him in order to reach a diagnosis.

In this somewhat detailed scenario you are given a pre-existing diagnosis and asked to make one for his abdominal pain, which must be related to the aneurysm. In answering your questions the patient will tell you that he was told that the main blood vessel in his tummy is dilated like a sac in one area, and that he needs to be monitored in case it gets bigger. He may even have been told of the danger that this sac may leak at some time in the future. An aneurysm of the abdominal aorta is often diagnosed incidentally on ultrasound and it may only become symptomatic and cause pain when it begins to leak or when it expands and causes compression of the adjacent structures.

History

Pain in the abdomen can be related to any abdominal organ, vessel, nerve, muscle or bone, and the range of possible questions is vast. In the short time allotted for history-taking, you must first confirm that this patient was told that he has an aneurysm of the abdominal aorta, and then establish a connection between it and the pain. This is important because if his aneurysm is leaking he will need to be admitted for urgent surgical intervention.

Questions

Mr Paterson, would you please tell me what exactly happened?

You say you developed a sudden ache in your tummy when you were gardening and it got worse despite taking painkillers. Where exactly do you feel this pain?

Do you have any pain in the back?

Does it throb?

Is it constant or does it come and go?

Does it spread anywhere else?

Did you feel anything else in your tummy?

You said you had some painkillers. Did they have any effect on your pain?

Has the pain got worse since it started?

Have you had any similar pains in the past?

Have you had any other symptoms such as sickness, fever, diarrhoea, or trouble with your waterworks?

You said you were told that you had a vascular sac in your tummy. What else did they tell you?

When and how did they find it?

How big did they say the sac was?

Do you have any other medical conditions such as diabetes mellitus, high blood pressure or heart trouble?

You are the SHO in the A&E room where you see Miss Osborne, a 28-year-old lady presenting with a whiplash injury sustained in a recent car accident. An X-ray of her neck shows no bony injury but she complains of pain in her neck. Please take a history from her and advise her.

A whiplash injury of the neck is caused by a violent hyperextension–hyperflexion of the cervical spine when a driver or passenger in a vehicle is subjected to sudden acceleration or deceleration. The patient will experience pain, stiffness, and some restriction of movement (because of the pain in the neck), all of which usually settle within a few days with physiotherapy and painkillers. However, in some cases the symptoms persist and may even become worse although there is no bony injury to account for them. In many of these cases the problem is complicated by associated factors such as a claim for compensation or underlying depression.

History

The examiner will be checking that you not only take a detailed history of the injury and the resulting symptoms, but that you also explore the surrounding circumstances with tact and some delicacy.

Questions

Hello, Miss Osborne. How are you feeling now?
Is the pain any worse since the accident?
Do you feel pain if you look sideways?
Would you tell me how it all happened?

You say you were driving your car and suddenly found yourself
in a ditch. Forgive me for asking this, but was your mind
preoccupied in any way before the accident?

I am sorry to hear that you had had a double shock, losing your
job and your boyfriend a few days before the accident. Are you
feeling low in spirits?

Do you feel as interested in your hobbies or interests and social
life as you did before these events?

How do you sleep? Do you find it difficult to go to sleep or do
you wake up too early in the mornings?

Do you feel miserable and cry sometimes?

Are you looking for another job now?

Counselling

Doctor: Miss Osborne, you have sustained a whiplash injury to
your neck caused by a violent and unexpected movement of the
neck. There is no bony injury but the sudden jolt has caused
some minor damage to the soft tissues, giving you pain and
stiffness. I will give you some painkillers for the pain, and you
will need to increase the movements in your neck gradually. I
will arrange for you to see our physiotherapist who will give you
some massage and exercise. These symptoms should settle within
a few days, but I'm afraid quite a large part of the problem is that
you are depressed, which is quite understandable after what you
have gone through recently. You will need to restart your life and
look for another job, although I appreciate that this is easier said
than done. If the depression gets worse, then we may have to
consider a session or two with a psychiatrist. Is that all right?

Miss Osborne: Yes, doctor. Thank you.

Counselling and communication

Introduction

Counselling and effective communication are the 'return loop' of history taking, and should be just as professional, compassionate and sensitive. These days, when patients expect and demand to know more, and when the emphasis is on getting the patients to participate in the decision-making process, it is more important than ever to keep them informed at every stage. It is difficult to involve patients in their management unless they are kept well informed about their illness and treatment. If a patient is asked to give consent for a procedure then he must understand what is going to take place; the possible benefits resulting from that procedure; the consequences of not having the procedure; and the possible complications that may arise from it.

Unfortunately, until recently communication skills were not part of the medical curriculum and were not taught as a subject anywhere. Doctors learned communication by a process of osmosis as they went along, on ward rounds or sitting in as students in outpatient clinics. This inevitably left many gaps in the communication skills of younger clinicians; the older ones tended to learn from their own and others' mistakes. This hit-or-miss strategy has created a bad impression with the public and the media, and has lately tarnished the good image of the medical profession. The professional bodies as a whole, however, have now undertaken to put their house in order. One inescapable consequence has been the inclusion of communication skills both in learning and assessment in medical teaching. As a result of an increasing emphasis on communication and counselling, there will be at least three OSCE stations where the spotlight will be on communication skills.

As in the history-taking stations, you will be given 1 minute to read and grasp the instruction outside the station. On the bell you will go in and find a 'patient' (usually an actor or actress), with whom you will interact while the examiner looks on. The instruction will spell out clearly what you have to do (e.g. tell a patient, or his relative, that he has cancer; get consent for an operation). The actor will have a printed sheet telling them what they are supposed to do and say and the examiner will also have a printed mark sheet telling him what to look for. The 'patient' or 'relative' may be aggressive, aggrieved, or upset, but be reassured they will not become violent or lose their temper with you! It is your job to soothe their ruffled feathers or console them, and communicate the information with compassion and sensitivity.

There are four golden rules you must observe which apply whenever you are going to inform somebody about something of which he has either no knowledge or only partial knowledge:

1. *Find out how much the other person knows and their level of understanding.* It is impossible to build anything unless you know the bottom line and where to build. The preliminary chat is made easier by such enquiries, and it may only take one question to assess a person's conversational ability as well as his knowledge of the subject. If you don't know what the other person knows, the conversation can become turgid and your listener may become suspicious that you are hiding something behind your jargon and big words.

2. *Develop a dialogue.* It is bad practice to give long chunks of information without allowing the listener time to digest and ask questions for clarification. The listener may also conclude that you do not care and want to be finished as soon as possible. A useful way of generating responses is to pause at strategic moments, when you feel that the listener may want to ask a question or offer some comment. Good conversationalists often give information in small bits, stopping after every two or three bits to solicit questions.

3. *Give bad news with compassion and sensitivity.* Apart from the obvious fact that bad news should be given with some evidence of feeling, it is important to find something optimistic to add to make the news a little less painful. A simple rule of thumb is to find a 'but' to accompany every piece of bad news. For example, after telling a patient that he has a lymphoma, you may have to expand, 'Yes, you are right that lymphoma means cancer of the lymph glands, *but* there are several treatment options available to us.' The purpose here is not to give a falsely positive picture, or create unrealistic expectations, but rather to find something comforting and hopeful to say when you are conveying bad news. You must be mindful of your body language and appear sympathetic when you mean to console. Impart warm, tactile solace with a firm handshake, and offer a cup of tea and a box of tissues if required.

4. *Offer opportunities for further enquiries and sources of further information.* Hearing unpleasant news is often such a shock

that it renders patients unable to take in any detailed information. A patient who has just been told that she has diabetes mellitus, for example, may be too shocked to grasp the fine details of the condition, and a lecture on the apparently trivial subject of foot care would be a waste of time. It is also human nature to look for a second opinion that would be more positive than the one just received. Most people given information about a sinister condition, about their lifestyle, or about the future management of a condition, feel suffocated between time and information. They need time to breathe freely and to think things out logically for themselves, and would then need access to someone to ask more questions. For all these reasons it is important to offer further opportunities to ask questions; information leaflets they can read at leisure; and the addresses of agencies which can offer more information and support.

In this section, we have presented 32 counselling and communication scenarios which are commonly encountered in clinical practice and in exams. The exact format of presentation of these cases was a source of a great deal of anxiety and uncertainty but after discussions with many doctors who had already passed their PLAB examination, we settled on the conversational style. There are two compelling reasons for this. First, information about the various subjects in Section 3 is available in many books and simply reproducing it here would be little comfort to those candidates whose main problem is that they are unfamiliar with spoken English. Second, in the exam you may be asked to tackle only one or two aspects of a subject and the conversational format allowed us to break a large subject into small chunks. This format also allows you space to encourage the patient or relative to ask you questions. You will need to practise with a colleague to improve your style in this regard.

Alison Fisher, a 16-year-old girl, has recently developed acne on her face for the first time. She is very worried about it and wants some treatment to clear it up and also advice about how to prevent it coming back. She is particularly concerned about the possibility of scars. You are her GP and you haven't seen her for some time as she is usually very healthy. Please talk to her.

Acne in young women causes a lot of distress, both physical and psychological. Acne can be unpleasant and can easily disrupt social life, particularly in teenagers. When you talk to this young lady you should sympathize and reassure her. She may want to ask you about the following issues:

- What causes acne?
- What can be done to control/cure it?
- Will there be any scars?
- Are there any lifestyle changes that might help?
- Can the oral contraceptive pill make it worse?

Doctor: Good morning, Miss Fisher. How can I help you?

Miss Fisher: I am very concerned about the spots on my face. Can you tell me why I've got them and what I can use to get rid of them?

Doctor (*after examining the face*): OK. These spots are acne or, as some people call them, teenage spots. They usually occur in young people because their skin is abnormally sensitive to a chemical called androgen circulating in the body. It is very common at your age. This chemical, which is a hormone, causes the skin to produce more oil and so it becomes greasy, especially

over the face, back, and shoulders. There are special glands in
your skin called sebaceous glands that produce oily secretions.
The pores in these glands become blocked with these sticky, oily
secretions which then can't escape and the glands swell up and
form acne spots. Often some bacteria collect in the glands, act on
the oil, and release chemicals that irritate the surrounding skin
even more. It is rather like trying to pour oil out of a balloon
with a long thin neck — when the neck is blocked the oil builds
up in the balloon.

Miss Fisher: What can be done to sort it out?

Doctor: Well, in your case the acne is not severe and we should
be able to control it. I will prescribe an ointment that you will
need to use regularly. This ointment reduces the amount of
bacteria, or infection, and unblocks the pores in the skin, and so
helps the acne to heal up. See how this treatment goes for the
next few weeks. You should find that the spots gradually
disappear. When you see any new spots forming, start to use the
ointment again before they get too big. This will reduce the risk
of them leaving any marks. Try not to pick them, however
tempting that is — picking them just spreads the bacteria
around, makes the inflammation worse, and increases the risk of
scarring.
　Keep your skin clean with ordinary soap and water. You don't
have to use medicated soaps. Any of the cleansing lotions that
are available in most chemists can be useful.

Miss Fisher: What about diet?

Doctor: That is a good question. Although we know that special
diets do not *prevent* acne, it is important that you maintain a
healthy, balanced diet. You *can* eat sweets, fruit, and even
chocolate — you will probably hear older people in your family
tell you that the spots are due to too many sweets, but this is not
so!

Miss Fisher: What if the acne gets worse?

Doctor: If the acne gets worse, there are other medical treatments
that might help. Stronger ointments are available and sometimes
we also use a course of antibiotics to control the infection in the

spots and to speed up healing. If we need more help after that I would refer you to a dermatologist.

Miss Fisher: I am on the 'pill', doctor. Can I keep taking it?

Doctor: Oral contraceptive pills can sometimes cause a skin reaction but it does not make acne worse. In fact, there is a preparation containing oestrogen as well as an anti-androgen, co-cyprindiol, that is especially prescribed for women with severe acne. Remember, it is the androgen that causes the trouble.

Miss Fisher: Will the acne go away completely?

Doctor: Yes, you will grow out of it in time. There are, however, no easy solutions and you will no doubt find that spots will appear on and off for some time. If your acne does get worse we will try different ointments, antibiotics, and other drugs, like the one I mentioned. As you get older the acne will become less troublesome and it will gradually disappear.

I know that these teenage spots can be quite uncomfortable and sometimes embarrassing. Don't let it stop you doing all the things you want to do. Many, many teenagers get this and they all have to get on with life. Many of your friends will have them at some stage. Is there anything else you would like to ask me?

Miss Fisher: Oh yes, I nearly forgot. I read recently somewhere that there is a wonder drug called 'mino-something-line' but it has side-effects. Could you tell me something about it.

Doctor: I haven't read the article you mentioned but it sounds like minocycline, which is an antibiotic used for treating various infections and acne. It does have many side-effects and can affect almost any organ of the body, particularly the hearing, balance, the liver and the kidney. It also interferes with other drugs you might be on, including penicillin and the oral contraceptive. However, as I said, if you need more powerful drugs then we will get you seen by a dermatologist who will be happy to explain everything.

In the meantime, try this cream. Come back if you feel you need to try another preparation for your skin. Come back when your supply runs out or if you are worried.

Mr King, a 46-year-old man, is being discharged from hospital after recovering from an episode of alcoholic hepatitis. You are the SHO in the team. Explain to him the harmful effects of alcohol, and advise him to stop drinking in order to prevent any further, and possibly more serious, damage to his liver.

When talking to this patient, find out first what he knows about alcohol abuse and its effects, whether he has considered or tried giving up the habit, and what, if anything, makes him drink. Explain to the examiner that you would have done this while you had been treating him in hospital. You should explore further with him the potential harmful effects of alcohol and stress the potential benefits of abstinence.

If you were talking to a female patient you should also explain that alcohol affects fertility and it can damage unborn babies. Also, because women can get drunk more easily than men, their personal safety may be jeopardized.

Counselling a heavy drinker needs some experience as well as knowledge. This may be a difficult scenario for you if you have lived and worked in a country where alcohol is not permitted due to religious beliefs. You may not have had any first hand experience. Examiners are not after your knowledge as much as they are testing your communication skills here. They do expect you to be compassionate and polite and yet it is important for them to see how you would try to persuade a drinker, at risk of serious ill health, to come to terms with his addiction and to accept help.

Doctor: Good morning, Mr King. I am delighted to be able to tell you that you are ready to go home today.

Mr King: I can't wait, doctor.

Doctor: Fine. I understand that. Well, you have been in the hospital for over a week now. As you know, when you came in you were very ill. You had jaundice and you were confused and quite unwell. Tests showed that you had inflammation of the liver caused by alcohol, what we call alcoholic hepatitis. Abstinence, medication, and a few days' rest in the hospital have made you a lot better and your liver is recovering very well.

You have told me that you are essentially a beer drinker and that you drink about 8 pints a day, mostly at lunchtime and in the evenings.

Mr King: Yes, that is about it. I have been made redundant recently. There isn't much to do so I go out drinking at lunchtimes as well as in the evenings. I don't get drunk as such, though. (*Remember that heavy drinkers always underestimate the amount they consume.*)

Doctor: Mr King, I am sure you appreciate that you have been drinking well over five times the recommended limit in the last few months. The maximum for a man is 21 units, or 10 pints, per week — one unit is half a pint of beer. You are drinking about 16 units each day and this is well over 100 units per week. Are you aware what this excessive alcohol consumption is doing to you?

Mr King: Yes, doctor. I could see it coming and I know of some of the dangers but somehow I always think that it won't do me any harm.

Doctor: The most important thing to remember is that this problem with your liver is likely to happen again, and it will get worse, if you go back to your old drinking habits.

Mr King: Hmm … I know. I do want to give up but somehow I just keep going back to it.

Doctor: Just to make sure that we are talking about the same thing, let me go through some of the problems of alcoholism with you. Alcohol is like a drug with lots of side-effects. Excess alcohol consumption can damage literally every organ in your body. Your liver is already showing signs of damage and this may become permanent if you continue to drink. Cirrhosis, or permanent scarring of the liver, can be a very serious and life-threatening problem. Alcohol also makes you more likely to develop peptic ulcers, pancreatitis — which is an inflammation of the pancreas — and cancer of the oesophagus or stomach. Alcohol can affect your heart and increase your blood pressure. In fact, every pint of beer adds a few millimetres to your blood pressure. Alcohol can also cause serious damage to your brain and the nerves — it can cause memory problems, damage to the nerve endings, and psychiatric problems. Alcohol can also affect your sexual function. In fact, Mr King, the list is endless.

Think about the social effects as well. If you get a new job your performance at work could be affected and you are probably spending more money on drink than on anything else. You may get into trouble with the police because of the way you behave when you are drunk. If you drink and drive you are taking unnecessary risks with your own and others people's lives. Alcohol can ruin your family life too.

Mr King: It all sounds very grim, doctor.

Doctor: Yes, but it is never too late to stop. Mr King, have I given you enough reasons to stop drinking? I do understand that it is not easy to stop. However, if you really want to try then I believe you will be able to give up the habit. The strength of will power that you will need should come from wanting to prevent permanent damage to your health, and to your liver in particular — liver failure is always fatal. You will have taken the first step towards stopping drinking when you really believe that alcohol is bad for you. The benefits of giving up would be that your liver will recover, that there will be no further damage to other organs, and that you would have a healthier life style with spare cash to spend on the other things you would like to have.

Mr King: How can I get help, doctor?

Doctor: As I said, the first step is for you to believe that alcohol is bad for you. Once you have a sincere desire to get help, there are several ways of getting it. There are community 'drugs and alcohol' teams in every part of the country and there is one locally. These health care workers are specially trained in this field. You can refer yourself, or you can be referred through your

GP. We can also start the process from the hospital if you would like that. Once you have been referred you will have formal counselling by an expert and things will go on from there. Though it may sound complicated, believe me, once you get into the system you will get all the help you need.

Mr King: Does it work?

Doctor: Well, yes and no! It depends entirely on you. The more determined you are, the more likely it is that it will work. A significant proportion of patients remain alcohol-free for a long time. Believe me, it does work for many patients. Unfortunately, there are also many whose resolve does not last long, and one or more of their vital organs eventually succumb to the ravages of alcohol.

Mr King: OK. I will really have to think about this. I think if I could get back into a job it would help.

Doctor: Here is an information sheet that gives all the information that you need and also some useful phone numbers. You can also join 'Alcoholics Anonymous', where you would have the opportunity to meet other people who have been in a similar situation as yourself. They follow twelve well set out principles and a genuine desire to give up alcohol is the only qualification you need to join. Again, information about this is in the information sheet.

I hope you have found our discussion useful. Do you have any further questions?

Mr King: Yes. How could I start cutting down on the alcohol?

Doctor: Mr King, as I said before, you would need expert help. However, you might find some tips useful. The best strategy is to stop at once and I can give some medicine to help you during the withdrawal period. If you can't do that, then keep a drinking diary and adopt some personal drinking rules. Pace your drinking, sip slowly, take smaller sips, drink for taste, and do not mix beers with spirits. Try to be a slow drinker and put the glass down between sips. Tell your friends that you would like to buy your own drinks. Try spacer (spacing your drinks) instead of chaser (following one soon after another), dilute spirits, eat before drinking, and learn to refuse a drink. These tips may help you to gain some control over your habit, but your ultimate goal should be to stop drinking completely. Any other questions?

Mr King: No, not at the moment.

Doctor: Fine. Shall we see you in the clinic in 6 weeks, just to make sure that everything is all right? Also, we can monitor your progress and check this with regular blood tests of your liver function. There is a test which measures a substance in your blood called gamma-GT which will tell us if you have been drinking too much.

Mr King: Thank you, doctor.

Mr Bedford, a 68-year-old man, has been diagnosed as having Alzheimer's disease. He had been becoming increasingly forgetful over the last 6 months and eventually his son persuaded him to get some medical advice. You are the SHO on the elderly psychiatric assessment ward. Talk to Mr Bedford, his son (and his main carer) about what the future holds.

The diagnosis of Alzheimer's disease carries with it a lot of psychosocial implications, not only to the patients but also to their immediate family. Both patients and their carers need help and support. A clear explanation about the disease process and the likely clinical course should be explained to this patient's carer. This would enable him to come to terms with the problem and he would have a much clearer idea of what to expect in the future. In your discussion you should focus on the treatment options and support networks available for the patient. At the same time you should recognize that the carer also might need help and support himself.

Doctor: Good morning, Mr Bedford. I am Dr Khan. I know you are anxious to discuss your father's recent illness and all that has been going on over the last few months. Perhaps we can begin by you giving me some idea about what you understand about your father's condition. (*Listen to this carefully and then build on it to improve his understanding.*)

Mr Bedford: Thank you for taking the time to talk to me, doctor. (*He tells you what he knows so far.*)

Doctor: As you told me, your father has been behaving rather oddly for the last 6–8 months. He has been forgetful and depressed. He has been confused at times. We have performed several investigations including a CT scan of the brain. I'm afraid all these tests suggest that he has Alzheimer's disease. I'm sorry, I realise that it's no consolation to know the explanation for his behaviour.

Mr Bedford: I was afraid of that. It is a kind of dementia, isn't it?

Doctor: That's right. Alzheimer's disease is a type of dementia. It is a slowly progressive disease that affects all the functions of the mind over a period of several years. It reduces your ability to concentrate, remember and reason.

Mr Bedford: What causes it?

Doctor: Although the cause of Alzheimer's disease is not entirely known, we do know that there are several predisposing factors. They include genetic factors, or abnormalities in some chromosomes, increased levels of aluminium in the brain, and viral infections, to name but a few. Obviously, it is a very complex disease process and it ultimately leads to shrinking of the brain with loss of nerve tissue and an accumulation of what are called 'senile plaques' and 'neurofibrillary tangles'. Essentially, these cause changes in the levels of certain chemicals in the brain and are responsible for many of the symptoms of Alzheimer's disease.

Mr Bedford: Is it inherited? Will I get it?

Doctor: Though there is a definite genetic influence, it is not inherited in most patients. Some families have been described where this disease seems to be inherited. However, this is extremely rare.

Mr Bedford: Is his condition likely to deteriorate soon?

Doctor: Alzheimer's disease tends to be a slowly progressive disease. The rate of progression can be unpredictable. It is also hard to predict what problems or symptoms your father is likely to develop during the next few years. It is honestly a question of taking things as they happen. However, it is useful to know what problems your father might have in the future, so that you can be prepared for them. Memory loss is an early sign of Alzheimer's, as you know. This can get progressively worse. Your father may find it increasingly difficult to cope. He may find difficulty in expressing himself or in understanding others. He may get agitated or aggressive and may greatly overreact in certain situations. Ability to manage the activities of daily living, such as dressing, grooming and eating, decline throughout the illness. As the disease progresses he may wander, partly because he will have difficulty identifying his surroundings, and partly because of emotional difficulties. He may get increasingly confused or may develop psychiatric problems that would require specialist help.

Mr Bedford: What can I do to help my dad?

Doctor: OK. You can do a lot both for yourself and for your father by first accepting his illness. There are a few simple precautions that you can take to make things easier for him. Lock up any rooms in the house which are not used. Lock any drawers that contain important documents. Remove locks from the bathroom door, so that he cannot accidentally get locked in. While he can, get him into the habit of keeping a diary or using a dictaphone to remind himself about daily tasks. Make a list of things that he needs to do. Remind him about things frequently but be patient if he asks you the same question repeatedly. Let him talk about 'old times' — this will boost his morale, as memory for distant events remains intact long after the ability to recall recent events has gone.

Mr Bedford: What other help is available?

Doctor: Though it is not curable, a lot can be done to help patients and their carers. Your father will require a tailored package of care involving a multidisciplinary team that can provide support and advice. Social services offer many of these services. Care managers will carry out an assessment of the services that are needed to support him at home, including home care, personal care, meals on wheels, special equipment, mobility aids, financial advice, access to day centres, and access to residential or nursing care if that should be needed in the future. It is important therefore that you have contact with the social worker as soon as possible. Help at the right time can make all the difference.

Community nursing, physiotherapy if necessary, health visitors, and the continence adviser can be arranged through the hospital or your GP. Your GP can also refer your father to other specialists, such as the community psychiatric nurse, occupational therapist, psychologist, dietitian, psychiatrist and community health care assistants. Information about self-help groups and other voluntary organizations can be obtained through the social services or the local Citizen's Advice Bureau. All in all, these services should be able to look after the physical and psychological needs of your father.

Mr Bedford, looking after your father may be physically and emotionally exhausting and therefore you must look after yourself as well. Although initially you might like to do everything for your father, do make use of any help from family and friends that may be available. This will give you time to relax and recharge your batteries. Caring for your father will sometimes make you feel isolated, stressed, and frustrated. Feelings of guilt are very common in family carers and this can undermine your confidence. You must always remember that you are not to blame for having these feelings. You should see your GP regularly to discuss any problems and needs as they arise.

I strongly advise that you and your father join the local Alzheimer's Society. They provide information, advice, and support to people with dementia and their families. The services available include a helpline, carers' support meetings, and a members' newsletter. They hold branch meetings with talks about research and other topics and provide training for carers and professionals on how to understand and care for the person with dementia. If it becomes necessary, they also organize relief care in the home through partnership contracts with the Crossroads Care Scheme. As an organization they are important campaigners for individual person-centred care services.

Mr Bedford: Are there any benefits that we could claim?

Doctor: Benefits are available to patients with Alzheimer's disease and their carers. You should contact the Benefits Enquiry Line for advice. They will send you forms and help you to fill them in. You can also contact your local Benefits Agency or the local Citizen's Advice Bureau. You should make sure that you both get all the benefits and allowances available, including disability allowance for your father.

Mr Bedford: What about this new drug, Aricept, for Alzheimer's disease? I read about it in the papers recently.

Doctor: That's right. This drug is also called 'donepezil' and has been licensed in the UK. Clinical trials have shown a modest improvement, or delay, in the deterioration of mental function in patients with Alzheimer's disease. However, there are a lot of issues that still need to be answered before this drug becomes widely available. The first thing is that the drug is likely to be most beneficial if used in the early stages of the disease. The diagnosis of early Alzheimer's disease is very difficult and, as you know, most patients have gone beyond the early stage when they are diagnosed. We also do not know what would happen if the drug is stopped after long-term treatment. Lastly, the issue of when to stop treatment is a very difficult one both on clinical grounds and on ethical grounds. Because of all these unsettled issues, the Health Authority has not given us funding to use this drug at this stage. However, if it becomes available in the future, then certainly we should consider offering this treatment to your father. However, there are other drugs that can be given if any of the symptoms, such as depression or delusions, become troublesome.

   Mr Bedford, I'm afraid there is no single or simple solution and I can understand your anxieties. However, we are here to help you and your dad. Once you have made contact with the social worker and other support services, you will be able to access them whenever you need them and you can always get back to us. Is there anything else you would like to ask?

Mr Bedford: No, thank you.

Doctor: Take care.

Mr Seymour, a 20-year-old-man, has recently been admitted to hospital with severe breathlessness and has been diagnosed as having bronchial asthma. You are the medical SHO. Talk to him about this condition and what he needs to do to minimize problems in the future.

A diagnosis of asthma in a 20-year-old man will obviously cause considerable anxiety and you should give the patient ample opportunity to express this. The issues that you should address include explanations about:

- The nature of the problem
- The steps the patient can take to prevent an attack of asthma
- The use of the different inhalers
- How to deal with an attack of asthma at home

Doctor: Good morning, Mr Seymour. How are you today?

Mr Seymour: I am very well, thank you, and I'm looking forward to going home today.

Doctor: Naturally! Before you go, I'd better have a chat with you.

Mr Seymour: OK.

Doctor: As you know, you were admitted with sudden onset of breathlessness and cough over the weekend. You were quite wheezy at that time and tests have shown that you have bronchial asthma. This is a condition that affects the airways — the tubes that carry air in and out of the lungs. What actually happens is that your airways suddenly get narrowed, which makes you cough and feel breathless and a tightness in your chest.

Mr Seymour: What causes the narrowing of the airways?

Doctor: The airways have muscles in their walls which allow them to vary their calibre as the need arises. In asthma these contract, causing narrowing of the tubes. The inside of the tubes is inflamed and as a result there is swelling of the walls and a build-up of secretions which lead to further narrowing. This happens when you are exposed to trigger factors such as infections, smoke, pollen, and dust. It is a form of allergic reaction to these and many other substances.
Has anybody explained to you about inhalers?

Mr Seymour: Yes, but I am not sure about why there are different kinds.

Doctor: Well, inhalers can be used either to *treat* an attack or to *prevent* an attack. The blue ones, which contain salbutamol, are the relievers — that is, they help to deal with an attack. The brown ones, which contain steroids, are used to prevent an attack. You should use your inhalers as directed. You should be taking the brown inhaler twice a day, two puffs each time. The blue inhaler is to be used as and when your chest is tight. Take two puffs at a time but don't use it more than four times in a day. There are some side-effects if you use the blue inhaler too much — basically, you can become tremulous and get shaking fingers and hands, and you may feel your heart racing.

Mr Seymour: What can I do to prevent these attacks from happening again?

Doctor: There are several ways you can help yourself. You should try to maintain a healthy lifestyle. Take regular exercise, although you may find that very strenuous exercise can bring on some wheezing. Most important of all is that you should not smoke. A clean home will reduce your exposure to triggers — this means that you must ensure that your environment is as dust-free as possible because the house-dust mite lives in dusty environments and this is one of the main triggers for asthma. Vacuum-clean your mattress and shake out the blankets regularly. Avoid contact with cats and dogs and avoid aspirin and any tablets that contain it. Aspirin contains salicylic acid which is a well-known trigger. Avoid foods that you think might precipitate an attack — these will often be the ones that contain large amounts of salicylate, such as curries, herbs, spices, and mustard. You might find that cold air is a problem, particularly when out walking in the winter.

Mr Seymour: What do I do if I have an attack of asthma at home?

Doctor: If you feel that an asthma attack is about to come on, the first thing to do is to sit down and try to relax. Take two puffs of the blue inhaler. You should be all right in a few minutes. Sometimes, for example when you have a bad cold, you may find that you need to continue to use the inhalers for a bit longer, but never go above the recommended dose (i.e. 2 puffs, 4 times a day). If you are still wheezing or uncomfortable, or find that you are getting worse, you must call your doctor immediately. Does that answer your question?

Mr Seymour: Yes, thank you.

Doctor: Mr Seymour, I would now like to see how you use the inhaler and check on your technique. (*Allow him to demonstrate his inhaler technique.*)
   That was not too bad! However, let me show you the best way of using the inhaler. First, shake the inhaler. Breathe out fully. Place the mouthpiece of the inhaler between your front teeth and put your lips around the mouthpiece to form a seal. Press the canister once just as you begin to breathe in deeply through your mouth. After breathing in fully, hold your breath for about 10 seconds and then breathe out slowly.
   Do you want to have another go? (*Check whether he is doing it properly.*)
   You can get an idea of how severe an attack is, and of your progress, by using a peak flow meter, which is this little gadget. Breathe in fully and then blow into this mouthpiece as hard as you can (see p. 391). Your blow will be recorded on the meter in litres per minute. You can keep a daily record of your readings. This daily record will show you if your chest is getting tight — the peak flow readings would fall. Also, when you have an asthma attack, a rise in the reading will show if the treatment is working.
   Here is an information sheet on asthma that I thought you might find useful. There is a lot of information available on the

Internet and you could join the local Asthma Group. Is there anything else that you would like to ask me?

Mr Seymour: What about the other pills that I am taking at the moment? Some of these are steroids. Aren't they harmful if taken for too long?

Doctor: Take your medications regularly until they are finished, but you will need to tail off your steroid tablets gradually. When you take steroid tablets your body's ability to produce its own steroids is reduced. When you tail off steroids gradually your body has time to recover and produce its own steroids when these are needed. As described in the prescription, you will have to reduce the steroid dose by 10 mg each week.

I have made an appointment for you in our Asthma Clinic in 6 weeks' time. If you have any further questions or if you have any new problems, however, please do not hesitate to contact me.

David, a 9-year-old boy, has been diagnosed with atopic eczema. You are the paediatric SHO. Talk to Mrs French, his mother.

Atopic eczema is a common condition in children. It occurs most commonly in infancy and childhood and is much less common in adults. David obviously has the childhood form of atopic eczema. Mrs French may ask you some of the following questions:

- What is atopic eczema?
- Will it disappear?
- Is David likely to have any other problems?
- What is the treatment?
- Is there anything that we can do to prevent the eczema?
- Is it inherited?

Doctor: Good morning, Mrs French. As you know, David has had an itchy rash on his elbows, wrists, neck and his face for 3 to 4 weeks. We call this atopic eczema. It is a very common condition in childhood and David's rash is very typical. Do you have any idea what it means?

Mrs French: Atopic eczema? No, could you explain it?

Doctor: Well, atopic eczema is a skin condition which has developed because David reacts abnormally, and has an allergy, to certain substances in the environment, which are harmless to most children. This abnormal reaction shows up as eczema, which is a kind of skin rash.

Mrs French: What causes it?

143

Doctor: The cause of this is not entirely known. But we do know that the immune system, or the body's defence system, plays a crucial role. Some children's immune systems react abnormally to substances in the environment. Why the immune system reacts abnormally is not known but this tendency may be inherited. In fact, 70% of patients have a family history of asthma, hay fever, or dermatitis, all of which are allergic reactions.

Mrs French: What can be done to treat it, doctor?

Doctor: There is no sure way of curing this problem but we can do a lot to control the symptoms. Avoiding skin irritants is very important, the most common irritants being soap and hot water. David should bathe using warm — not hot — water. He should not apply too much soap to his arms and legs. Use an emulsifying ointment instead of soap and add Oilatum to the bath water. Applying a moisturizer and a steroid cream should help. Put the steroid cream onto the affected areas of skin once a day. You can use the moisturizer as and when necessary. Topical steroids are less likely to cause side effects than steroids in tablet form. However, used over long periods, there can be side-effects, including slower growth, weight gain and thinning of the bones. To keep his skin as supple as possible, try to avoid exposing him to extreme cold or wind. Woollen clothes also cause irritation. Use man-made fibre duvets instead of feather and down duvets.

I'm afraid David will be more prone to skin infections. If there are any signs or worries about him developing a skin infection you should contact your GP immediately. Watch out for any signs of pus or yellowish pimples which could indicate that he has an infection.

I'll give you a prescription for a skin cream which should be applied three times a day.

Mrs French: What about food?

Doctor: Eczema is very rarely caused by foods in children and so we do not recommend any particular diets. However, there are other things that you can do. Keep the bedroom as free of dust as possible, vacuum-clean the mattress and wash the blankets regularly. Also, David should avoid contact with cats and dogs.

Mrs French: Will he always have this skin disease?

Doctor: No. David will almost certainly grow out of it in due course.

Mrs French: Will he be more prone to other problems, like asthma?

Doctor: Children with atopic eczema are at risk of developing asthma later. It is, however, difficult to measure that risk accurately. If both parents have an atopic condition then the chances are that it may also affect their children in later life. Mrs French, you should encourage David to lead a normal life as a child. Let him play with his friends and go to school as usual. Some precautions may be needed when going swimming. It is essential that David accepts this skin problem as part of life and does not feel that he is odd in any way. That way, he won't get any trouble from the other children at school with teasing or bullying.

Here is an information sheet giving you details about the National Eczema Society and some useful Internet sites. If you have any further questions please feel free to ask. How about coming back in a fortnight so that I can check that the skin is improving?

Mrs French: Thank you, doctor.

Doctor: Take care. Bye, Mrs French.

Talk to Matthew, a 7-year-old boy, before taking blood for investigations. He has been admitted with fever and headaches. You are the SHO on the paediatric ward and his mother is in the room with him.

To convince a 7-year-old boy to let you take blood can be a testing job for an SHO in paediatrics! This is usually done by trained paediatric phlebotomists, who would have a play therapist in with them to amuse and distract the child. In this case, the examiner is essentially testing your communication skills and your competence with the language. You should be friendly and honest with the child (i.e. don't say it won't hurt) and persuade him to have the blood test. You will need to be firm as well as kind.

Matthew will be understandably anxious and therefore will not absorb much information, but he will want to know if the test is really necessary and if it is going to hurt. In your conversation with him, you should bear in mind three important points. First, explain as simply as possible the need for the blood test and what it will achieve. Second, state outright that you are going to have to use a needle, but reassure him that you will use a spray or a cream which will minimize the pain. Third, suggest a subtle challenge which Matthew would be inclined to accept. For example, you could tell him that the needle you will use will be the smallest, a butterfly, which you use even on babies.

Doctor: Hi, Matthew, I am Rabia, your doctor. Are you all right?

Matthew: Hmm … I think so. But my head is sore.

Doctor: That is because you have a fever. You have been feeling hot, haven't you?

Matthew: Yes. What are you going to do?

Doctor: Well, the fever and sore head are probably caused by a bug that has got into your body. We need to know what bug it is so that we can give you the right medicine for it. Do you understand?

Matthew: Yes, I think so. How will you find out what bug it is?

Doctor: The bug has got into your blood and I will need a small amount of your blood to test it.

Matthew: Blood tests! Needles and stuff!?

Doctor: Yes, but I am going to use the smallest needle there is. Here, this is called a butterfly — see how small its point is? This is the one I use on small babies and it doesn't hurt much. Besides, I am going to use a special spray which will make the skin numb, and it will only hurt a tiny bit. As I said, I do the same on babies. (*Ethyl chloride spray can be used immediately before venepuncture, but tetracaine (amethocaine) gel has to be applied about 30 minutes before and should be wiped clean afterwards.*)
   You don't need to watch — you can talk to your Mum while I do it or you can watch it if you want to. Whichever way you like it. All right?

Matthew: OK, let's try the spray.

Doctor: Great. Let's get on then. Now Matthew, which side would you prefer?

Matthew: This one, please.

Doctor: OK. I am going to tie this special elastic band (*tourniquet*) around your arm while your Mum holds it for me, find a nice vein, spray over it and then clean the skin with these wipes. I will then gently put this needle in to get some blood.
   (*To Mum*) Are you all right holding his arm or would you rather not watch?
   OK. Here we go … Well done!

Mrs Jordan, a 46-year-old lady, had a right mastectomy for breast cancer a year ago. She has been readmitted with lethargy, vomiting, and weight loss. She now has metastatic disease with liver and lung secondaries. You are the SHO on the oncology ward. Talk to her about the diagnosis and prognosis.

Talking to this patient about the diagnosis might be very difficult. The examiners are testing not only your communication skills but also how compassionate and empathetic you are. Mrs Jordan is likely to have had chemotherapy and radiotherapy after the initial surgery. You have to be absolutely honest with her. Try not to give too much information all at once. She is not going to take it all in at this time.

Most patients who have been diagnosed as having cancer a year ago tend to be suspicious that it may have recurred, although there will be a few who are in denial to some extent and do not want to know the bad news. Answer her questions in simple language and avoid medical jargon. It is advisable to discuss the prognosis only if the patient wishes to do so. You should sound optimistic and hopeful.

All patients with cancer are usually on oncology follow-up rather than on general medical follow-up. Although the specifics of treatment are beyond the scope of this counselling session it is always useful to have some idea about treatment options and potential side effects.

Doctor: Good morning, Mrs Jordan. How are you doing today?

Mrs Jordan: I am feeling much better, doctor, thank you. Do you have the results of my scans and blood tests?

Doctor: Yes, I do. The results do show some abnormalities. As you know, when you came in last week you were complaining of a tickly cough, weight loss, and poor appetite. The blood tests have shown that your liver function is slightly disturbed and the chest X-ray shows some suspicious-looking shadows. You then had a CT scan of the chest and abdomen. I'm afraid it doesn't look very good. (*pause*)

Mrs Jordan: It's the same problem that I had last year, isn't it?

Doctor: I'm afraid so. Unfortunately, the scan shows that the breast cancer has spread to your lungs and liver, but there are some treatments available.

Mrs Jordan: What treatments are we talking about here?

Doctor: After the surgery last year you had chemotherapy and radiotherapy. Unfortunately, despite this the cancer has come back in the lungs and the liver. This means that we need to think about more chemotherapy to stop it spreading any further.

Mrs Jordan: Will the chemotherapy get rid of the cancer?

Doctor: There is a good chance that the chemotherapy would shrink the cancerous growths in the lungs and the liver. However, I don't think that it is going to be possible to get rid of the cancer completely. Some patients do go into complete clinical remission, by which I mean that the scans would be clear after treatment. It is impossible to predict who is going to respond well, and who is not, until the treatment is well under way, I'm afraid.

Mrs Jordan: Is this terminal? How long have I got?

Doctor: As I said, it is bad, but not that bad. In any case, I honestly do not know. However, what I can certainly tell you is that the chemotherapy has a very good chance of controlling the cancer for a reasonable period. There may also be the possibility of having some more radiotherapy in the future, if need be. As you can see, there are things that we can do to keep it under control. In many clinical trials patients have survived for anything from several months to a few years. There is also a lot of research going on in this field and newer treatments are being developed all the time.

Mrs Jordan: What chemotherapy am I going to have?

Doctor: As you have already had one lot of chemotherapy, the next step would be to give you docetaxel, a drug that your cancer cells have not been exposed to before. (*The choice of first-line chemotherapy for metastatic breast cancer depends on several factors, including: initial drugs used in adjuvant chemotherapy; age and performance status of the patient; initial histopathology and immunohistochemistry of the tumour; and underlying medical problems. Discussion about this would be beyond the scope of this counselling station.*) This chemotherapy tends to be an outpatient form of treatment. This means that you would need to come to the clinic once every 3 weeks to have the injections. The drug is given in an intravenous drip over 1 hour. We would give you at least three cycles of treatment (that is, three injections) and then repeat the scans. If everything is going in the right direction, then you will have a further three cycles of treatment.

Mrs Jordan: What are the side effects of this treatment?

Doctor: The side effects are likely to be similar to the ones that you had during your first lot of chemotherapy. Chemotherapy can give you nausea and vomiting. But we have very strong anti-sickness medications to control these symptoms. Chemotherapy is also likely to cause hair thinning and hair loss. Although this tends to be temporary, you could try scalp cooling to reduce the risk of hair loss.

Mrs Jordan: Scalp cooling did not work for me before. I think I will go for the wig again.

Doctor: That is fine. Chemotherapy can also give you a sore mouth, heartburn, tummy pains, and diarrhoea or constipation. Much more importantly it can drop your blood counts and make you more prone to infections. We would have to check your blood count regularly. Chemotherapy can also make you feel extremely tired. Docetaxel can cause an allergic reaction in some patients but we reduce the risk of this happening by giving you an injection before the chemo. All the information you need about chemotherapy is in this information sheet, Mrs Jordan. Have a careful read through it over the next few days.

Mrs Jordan: What if the chemotherapy does not work?

Doctor: If this drug does not work then we would need to think about further options. This will depend on what symptoms you have. As I said before, radiotherapy may be an option. We may also need to think about a different *form* of chemotherapy.

Mrs Jordan: What else can I do to help myself? What about diet?

Doctor: It is very important that you have a healthy and balanced diet. You must try to remain as positive and optimistic as possible. Many patients find alternative therapies very useful. There are also a lot of organizations that can help you through your illness, such as CancerBACUP. I can give you information sheets on these if you are interested. Many patients also find input from a Macmillan nurse extremely helpful. She can visit you at home and give you a lot of support and help. If you would like to go for this then I can talk to your GP and arrange it.

Mrs Jordan: Yes, I would like to have some more information. Can I think about the Macmillan nurse and get back to you over the next few weeks. When would I start treatment?

Doctor: OK. I would like to start the treatment within the next week or two. Can I arrange for you to see Karen again, our chemotherapy nurse, before you go home? She could go through the practicalities of the treatment with you. In the meantime I will get the information sheets for you. Please do not hesitate to contact us over the next few days if you have any questions.

Talk to Mrs Clark about breastfeeding. She is 30 weeks pregnant and undecided as yet about how she will feed the baby. You are the SHO in the antenatal clinic.

You may have to address several issues here, including:

- The advantages of breastfeeding (to the baby and to the mother)
- How breast milk is produced
- How long to continue breastfeeding
- The mother's diet during breastfeeding
- Problems associated with breastfeeding
- Where to find further information and help

Doctor: You are now about 30 weeks pregnant and we need to discuss how you are planning to feed the baby. Have you been thinking about breastfeeding?

Mrs Clark: What are the advantages of breastfeeding?

Doctor: You would be giving the best possible start in life to your baby by breastfeeding. Breast milk is a naturally designed food and contains all the necessary nutrients that your growing baby needs. Nature has designed breast milk in such a way that it can be easily digested and absorbed by your baby. Breastfed babies have fewer bowel infections, and less diarrhoea and constipation than bottlefed babies. Breast milk gives the baby resistance to infections like coughs and colds, and viral tummy troubles. This is because breast milk contains, in the form of antibodies, all the defences that you have built up over the years against infections. Eczema and other allergies are also less likely if your baby is breastfed.

Having gone through 9 months of pregnancy, many mothers feel that breastfeeding reinforces the closeness and bonding between the mother and the child after birth. You see, breast milk is readily available and costs nothing — you do not have to bother about preparing feeds or sterilizing bottles and equipment and your baby does not have to wait long when he or she is hungry. By the way, what would you like, a boy or a girl?

Mrs Clark: I don't mind, doctor, as long as the baby is healthy.

Doctor: And you can maintain that good health both for you and your baby by breastfeeding. It will also help you to lose some of the weight you will have put on during pregnancy, and your womb will get back to its normal state more quickly. Breastfeeding works as a form of natural contraception, particularly if no supplemental bottles are being given to the baby. However, you wouldn't be able to rely 100% on this and you should seek further advice from your midwife or GP.

Mrs Clark: How is the milk produced?

Doctor: This is a very complex process. During pregnancy, a lot of chemical changes happen in your body. These chemicals affect the breast tissue (glands and ducts) and prepare them for milk production. They are also responsible for the increase in the size of the breasts. During the first few days after the delivery of the baby the breasts produce a special discharge called colostrum. This is creamy and sometimes yellow in colour. It contains important nutrients your baby needs, including the antibodies that prevent infections.

After about 3 days or so, the milk becomes thinner. The milk that the breasts produce then can be divided into two types. The *fore-milk* that the baby takes first is thirst quenching, that is, it gives your baby the fluids he requires. The *hind-milk* that comes next provides the nutrition. As you can see, breast milk is indeed well designed and tailored for your baby's needs. The amount of milk produced will depend on the amount your baby feeds. That is to say, the more you breastfeed your baby, the more milk your breasts will produce. There is a message circuit, or reflex, from the nipple to the inside tissues of the breast. When the baby sucks on the breast, it produces the reflex. This causes the milk to collect behind the nipple, ready to flow.

Mrs Clark: What can I eat during breastfeeding?

Doctor: Breastfeeding is very thirsty work, so a healthy and balanced diet is very important. Make sure you drink a lot of extra fluids. Your body needs adequate vitamin D at this time. Eggs, milk, oily fish and fortified margarines are some of the foodstuffs that contain vitamin D. Your skin can make this vitamin when exposed to sunlight but make sure you use sunscreens to avoid sunburn.

Alcohol can get into the breast milk, so try to avoid it as much as possible. If there is any history of hay fever, eczema or asthma in your family (that is you, your partner, or your other children) avoid eating foods that may contain peanuts or peanut products. This precaution may reduce the risk of your baby acquiring a serious allergy to peanuts. If you find that some foods you eat upset the baby you should avoid eating them again. Also, you should not take any medications without prior discussion with your GP.

Mrs Clark: How long can I breastfeed?

Doctor: Breastfeeding for at least 4 months would be of great benefit. After that you can gradually wean the baby off milk and introduce semi-solids or liquidized chicken, meat, fish, or vegetables. If possible you could continue to give supplementary breastfeeding up to the baby's first birthday. Even if you switch to formula feeds you can still continue to breastfeed once or twice a day. Your midwife or health visitor can teach you how to go about breastfeeding your baby.

Mrs Clark: What problems might I have with breastfeeding?

Doctor: Breastfeeding can be a very fulfilling experience. However, if you are not aware of the possible difficulties during breastfeeding you may experience frustration and anxiety. Your breasts can get engorged during the first few days after delivery. This can be uncomfortable. Some mothers find a supporting bra helpful. Moreover, as you breastfeed you will notice that the engorgement settles down. Sore or cracked nipples is a common problem during breastfeeding. This can lead to infection and so you should get advice from your midwife or your GP. There are a few things you can do to avoid sore nipples, however: keep them dry as much as possible, avoid washing them after every feed, and avoid using soap. Change your breast pad frequently if necessary.

Lumpy, tender breasts are a common problem as well. Your midwife will advise you if this happens. It is caused by the milk ducts in your breast becoming blocked. If this happens let the baby feed on the tender breast first and gently massage the lumpy area with your fingertips to try and push the milk towards the nipple.

Mastitis, or bacterial infection of the breast, can make you unwell with fever, malaise, and pain in the breast. You would have to get help from your midwife or GP. You may require antibiotics for your mastitis but you should continue to breastfeed.

Your baby may feed restlessly. One of the possible reasons could be that the baby may be sucking too superficially at the nipple and may not be getting enough milk, or you may not be feeding your baby in the right position. When the baby feeds, she may be taking in some air as well. After the feed, sit up the baby on your knee and gently rub her back. This will help her to bring wind up. Sometimes, a little milk is brought up at the same time — this is called 'posset' and is entirely normal. If you have any problems you can always get help from your midwife or health visitor.

Mrs Clark: Where can I get some more information?

Doctor: As I said, you can get help and information from your midwife or the health visitor. Breastfeeding counsellors can be very helpful and the National Childbirth Trust can also provide you with valuable information. You can also join the Association of Breastfeeding Mothers. Here is an information sheet that gives you the addresses and contact phone numbers for these organizations. I trust you and your partner have already started going to parenting classes, which will prepare you for labour and the arrival of your baby. You will get more information about breastfeeding in these classes.

Above all, remember that breastfeeding is something that only you, as your baby's mother, can provide. Breastfeeding will provide your baby with the very best possible nutritional start in life, and give you as a proud new mother an emotional and loving bond with your new baby. It can be a great source of pleasure and joy and give you a great feeling of fulfilment.

Mrs Little, a 32-year-old lady, has had a cervical smear and the result is positive (i.e. it shows moderate dyskaryosis). You are the SHO in the department of obstetrics and gynaecology. Talk to her about the result and what it means.

In most centres in the UK, the results and recalls are sent to patients direct from a designated cervical-smear screening centre. In some circumstances a GP or someone in the gynaecology outpatients department may arrange follow-up. The counselling you offer would differ for the different categories of abnormality (normal cervical smear, inflammatory, mild atypia, mild dyskaryosis, severe dyskaryosis, invasion suspected, or abnormal glandular epithelium) and you should read up current recommendations in any of the major gynaecology textbooks.

This lady is likely to be anxious about the results. She would need to be reassured, whether the test is positive or negative. As the test is positive you will need to anticipate and answer the following questions:

- What does a positive test mean?
- Is it cancerous?
- What needs to be done about it?

Doctor: Good afternoon, Mrs Little. Please take a seat.

Mrs Little: Thank you, doctor.

Doctor: Well, you had your routine cervical smear a couple of weeks ago. I now have the result and I have to tell you that it is positive.

Mrs Little: What does that mean?

Doctor: It means that the smear showed some abnormal cells. Some of these look like the kind of cells that would have been on your cervix when you were developing in your mother's womb, when they were growing and multiplying fast. As you know, the smear was taken from the lining of the cervix — the neck of the womb. Therefore the test has shown that there are some abnormal cells lining the neck of the womb.

Mrs Little: Does this mean that I have cancer?

Doctor: No, it does not necessarily mean that there is cancer or that these cells will change any further. But I'm afraid the other side of that coin is that these abnormal cells do have a tendency to change further, which puts you at a higher risk of developing cancer. These cells *can* change their appearance and become cancerous. This means that there is a risk that you may have what we call a 'precancerous' (or leading to cancer) abnormality in the neck of the womb.

Mrs Little: How can I know definitely whether I have this precancerous abnormality or not?

Doctor: I was coming to that. The next step is to find out more by doing a colposcopy at the hospital, which means looking at the cervix, or neck of the womb, directly and taking samples of the abnormal looking areas. The samples can then be looked at under the microscope to see if there is any early cancerous change, such as cervical intraepithelial neoplasia. For short, this is also called 'CIN'. It can be of three types: I (mild), II (moderate), or III which is high-grade or severe. The higher grade type is more likely to become an invasive cancer. Grade III CIN is also known as 'carcinoma-in-situ', which means cancer confined to one limited area. There are various options available for treatment of CIN, including laser, cold coagulation, or electrodiathermy. I will explain these options more fully if the need arises. As I said earlier, a positive smear does not mean that you *definitely* have cancer, but it does mean that you are at a higher risk for developing it. So the next step is to have a biopsy as I explained earlier.

Mrs Little: When will I have the colposcopy?

Doctor: An appointment has been made for you to have the colposcopy in about 2 weeks' time. Here is an information sheet explaining the procedure. All the staff in the Colposcopy Unit are highly skilled in this examination and will explain the procedure as it happens. They are very sympathetic and understand that ladies are a little worried about this test. It is very important to have this abnormality investigated and treated at this stage. As doctors, we are always concerned that abnormal cells may develop into true cancerous cells if they are not treated. Fortunately, in this day and age we have an excellent screening service and the incidence of cervical cancer is dropping dramatically. Is there anything else you would like to ask me?

Mrs Little: Not at the moment, thank you, but I shall probably want to know more after this next test has been done.

Stephen, a 10-year-old boy, has recently been diagnosed with coeliac disease. His mother, Mrs Francis, is obviously concerned about the implications of such a condition in a child so young. You are the paediatric SHO and need to see her and explain all about the condition, answer her questions, and reassure her as much as possible.

Stephen's mother will need to understand the cause, effects, and treatment of coeliac disease. She needs to be reassured that her son will grow normally with appropriate treatment. She needs to be advised particularly with regards to the diet. The examiner will check whether you can address these issues.

Doctor: Good afternoon, Mrs Francis. I would like to explain to you about Stephen's recent problems and how we can treat him. If at any point during the conversation you have any questions please do not hesitate to ask.

Mrs Francis: Thank you, doctor.

Doctor: Well, as you know, Stephen has been losing weight for the past 6 months — not that he could really afford to lose any as his weight has always been on the low side. He has had occasional bouts of loose stools. You have also been worried that he has not been growing as tall as other boys of his age.
   Stephen has had a lot of tests in the last few days, including putting a tube down into his tummy. I know he did not particularly like that, but the tissue samples that we were able to take from his upper bowel have given us the answer to his problems. Sam has coeliac disease.

Mrs Francis: What does that mean?

Doctor: It is a condition affecting the small bowel in which the little villi, or outshoots, in the lining of the gut become flattened and so food isn't absorbed properly through the bowel wall. This causes malabsorption, or incomplete absorption, of nutrients and vitamins. What doesn't get absorbed goes straight down the bowel and causes the diarrhoea. What *does* get absorbed is insufficient for proper weight gain and growth. Here, let me explain it on a piece of paper. (*It would be a good idea to draw a simple picture for her, showing the villi and the route of absorption by means of arrows.*)
    Wheat, and wheat products like flour, contain a protein called gluten. Some people like Stephen can become intolerant to it, or to a part of the gluten called gliadin. Exactly why some people are intolerant to it is not entirely clear, but we do know that in some people gluten is not properly digested in the gut and that this can damage the lining of the small intestine. There is also some convincing evidence to suggest that the body's immune, or defence, system may be playing a crucial role in the development of coeliac disease. Some studies have suggested that some viral infections may possibly predispose to it. There is considerable debate about the actual cause. Be that as it may, the end result is that this damage to the lining of the gut means that Stephen is unable to absorb mainly fat and nutrients and this is the reason why he has lost weight, isn't growing properly, and has bouts of diarrhoea — whatever doesn't get absorbed just goes straight down the gut.

Mrs Francis: Is it inherited? Does Sam have abnormal genes?

Doctor: It is common to have more than one member of a family affected but the exact mode of inheritance is not known. About 1 in 10 of first-degree relatives tend to have the disease.

Mrs Francis: Is it treatable?

Doctor: Yes, it is certainly treatable. The majority of patients respond well to a gluten-free diet. In fact, many patients start feeling better within a few weeks of starting a gluten-free diet. I will explain to you in general what this diet involves and then Miss Sharp, our dietitian, will go through it in detail. She will give you a list of things that Stephen can and cannot eat. Basically, a gluten-free diet means eating no foods that contain wheat, rye, or barley flour. This would include bread, biscuits, cakes, and things like that. But do not worry. Stephen can make up for this by having enough milk, cheese, fruit, and vegetables. There is also a lot of processed food available that is specifically gluten-free. You can often substitute corn flour for wheat flour. You can buy special gluten-free bread from any health-food shop although most gluten-free foods can be bought in any supermarket as well as in specialist shops. Miss Sharp will go through all this with you in detail.

It is very important that Stephen sticks to a strict, and I mean a *really* strict, gluten-free diet. This will enable his weight and growth to catch up. On the diet his bowel will return to normal and eventually the absorption process returns to normal. Any slip in the diet, even a tiny amount of wheat flour, however, would mean a return of the diarrhoea.

Mrs Francis: Will he grow into a normal adult?

Doctor: There is no reason to believe that he will not do so. Most children with coeliac disease lead a normal life. They do catch up in height so he won't be compromised at all in terms of his growth. With a proper diet and support Stephen can achieve his full potential and I have no doubts about that.

Mrs Francis: Are my other children at risk? I have two daughters.

Doctor: Stephen's two sisters *will* be at a higher risk (1 in 10) than the general population, where the risk is 1 in 1500, for developing coeliac disease. Obviously you will need to keep that in mind, just in case. Look out for any similar symptoms, particularly the loose bowels, weight loss and tiredness. Remember also that they may not have the symptoms but still have the disease: your doctor will need to check them periodically for vitamin levels, such as folic acid and iron, in their blood. Is there anything else you would like to ask me?

Mrs Francis: No, thank you.

Doctor: I would like to see Stephen in 6 weeks' time to see how he is getting on with his new diet. Miss Sharp is going to see you and Stephen this afternoon. Can I also pass on this information sheet about coeliac disease? I am sure you will find it very useful. It also advises you on how to organize your holidays and eating out-of-doors. You could also consider joining the British Coeliac Disease Society.

Goodbye Mrs Francis, and take care.

Paul is a 7-year-old boy. He was recently admitted to hospital with weight loss, tiredness, and increasing thirst. He was found to have diabetes mellitus. You are the SHO on the paediatric ward and you are to talk to Mrs Savage, his anxious mother, about the condition and about how it will affect him both now and in the future.

Childhood diabetes mellitus has significant implications for a child's physical and psychological well-being. Paul's mother is understandably anxious and is likely to raise the following issues:

- The cause of diabetes (i.e. why has it happened to *her* child?)
- Treatment options
- Possible long-term effects and how to prevent them
- Side-effects of treatment and how to manage them
- The inheritance of diabetes (i.e. are her other children at risk?)

Doctor: Good morning, Mrs Savage. I am Dr Chang, the Senior House Officer in paediatrics. I am delighted to be able to tell you that Paul is getting better. However, I do need to talk to you about his condition.

Mrs Savage: Thank you, doctor, for seeing me. Paul got ill so fast that I have not been able to understand how it all happened.

Doctor: That is understandable. As you know, Paul had been feeling tired for the last few weeks and had been losing weight. You mentioned when he came in that he had been very thirsty and passing a lot of urine. You also said that he had started bed-wetting, which was unusual for him. When he was admitted to hospital 2 days ago he was very dry and had lost a lot of body fluids. Blood tests showed that he had very high levels of sugar in his blood. The blood sugar level at any time should be less than 8 mmol/L and Paul's was 30 mmol/L. So you can see it was very high. This was the reason for his tiredness and why he was so dry. This high a sugar level in the blood makes you very thirsty and drink a lot of fluids. And when you drink more you also pass a lot more water, causing dehydration, or dryness in the body. Dehydration can make children very unwell.

Mrs Savage, these are the classic features of diabetes mellitus. Now, I realize that this will come as a big shock to you although you may have been wondering about this possibility. It is quite likely that you know someone with diabetes already and may be familiar with the symptoms.

Mrs Savage: Diabetes? My father had it. I thought it only happened in adults.

Doctor: Well, there are different types of diabetes mellitus. In general, type I diabetes happens in the young and type II diabetes in adults, though this is not always the case. Sugar is a readily usable energy and the liver makes it from the food we eat. This sugar gets to the various parts of the body in the bloodstream but it cannot get *inside* the cells, to be used, without a chemical called insulin which comes from a gland called the pancreas that lives behind the stomach. If the special cells in the pancreas are damaged then there will be little or no insulin, with the result that there will be an excess of sugar floating around which cannot be used. This state is called type I diabetes. The mechanism of the damage to these special cells is not entirely known. There may be a combination of factors that trigger the damage, and possibilities include genetic factors and viral infections. (*Pause and allow Mrs Savage to ask questions.*)

In older patients, it is mostly resistance to insulin that makes the available insulin ineffective causing the same problem of too much sugar that cannot be used, and this variety is called type II diabetes. Paul has type I diabetes.

Mrs Savage: What is the treatment?

Doctor: As the pancreas does not make enough insulin we have to give it by injection under the skin. Initially, Paul was so dry that he needed fluids through a drip and so we were able to give him insulin through that in order to control his sugar level fairly quickly. We are now starting insulin by injection, twice daily under the skin. The current dose and regimen of insulin is working very well and Paul's blood sugar levels are very much better.

Mrs Savage, injecting insulin like this is the only way of keeping his blood sugar under control. He will need at least twice daily injections now — long term. The frequency of injections may vary from time to time, depending on his blood sugar levels.

Mrs Savage: Who will give him the injections at home? I would be a bit worried about giving them myself.

Doctor: The diabetic nurse, Mrs Shaw, is going to talk to you today in detail about insulin injections. Paul is still very young and it would be safer if you could give him his injections every day until he learns to do it himself. I know the thought of giving injections to your son is not pleasant but, believe me, you will get used to it very quickly. Mrs Shaw will teach you how to give the insulin injections to Paul. She will teach you how to draw up the correct dose and where to give the injections. We have a Diabetes Centre in this hospital where there are group sessions and you will have plenty of opportunities to learn about diabetes and to meet other people who are in the same boat. Once Paul is old enough he will be taught how to administer his own insulin.

Mrs Savage: Is there anything else I need to know, doctor?

Doctor: Well, it is extremely important that Paul does not miss any of his meals. Missing a meal, particularly after an injection, will put him at risk of hypoglycaemia, which is a low blood sugar level that is harmful to the brain because the brain depends totally on sugar for energy. You must be able to recognize a 'hypo' because it can be very dangerous if it is not treated. In such a situation Paul may feel weak, hungry, sweaty, tremulous, and possibly irritable. He may feel faint. He may also feel sick or have tummy pains. Untreated hypoglycaemia can cause fits and unconsciousness. If at any time you think Paul is having a hypo give him sugary drinks, immediately, and take him to your GP or the accident and emergency unit of the nearest hospital straightaway if he doesn't recover quickly. You will be able to get dextrose tablets which are handy when a hypo starts. You will also be given pre-filled glucagon injections which release stored sugar from the liver and which you can give him if he has a very bad hypoglycaemic episode making him unconscious.

Don't worry if you don't retain all of this at this stage. Mrs Shaw will tell you more about it.

Mrs Savage: How do I know if the blood sugar levels are under control at home?

Doctor: Mrs Shaw will also teach you how to monitor the blood sugar level at home using a meter. This is what we call the 'BM' test. You have to perform this fairly regularly, say four times every other day if stable; every day if the blood sugar levels are not stable. If the blood sugar is out of control (in other words, consistently above 8 mmol/L or below 4 mmol/L) then you must get the advice of our diabetes educator nurse. I will give you a leaflet which has her direct telephone number. You should not change the insulin dose yourself ... well, not to begin with. You will find, though, as time goes on that you will get to know how and when to make minor alterations in the dose according to the BM results.

It is important to remember that Paul's requirement of insulin may increase if he has any illness like flu. Again, you should contact us for advice. This is important because infections can make diabetes worse very rapidly, causing a serious problem called ketoacidosis. This happens when there is a very high level of blood glucose and also of other chemicals in the body which can be dangerous if not corrected early.

Paul will be followed up regularly in the Diabetes Clinic. This is to ensure that he is maintaining optimal blood sugar control and this will help to prevent any of the long-term problems associated with uncontrolled blood sugar levels. You should keep in regular touch with Mrs Shaw and her colleagues in the Diabetes Centre who will advise you from time to time. They will also talk with Paul. Children are always very keen and quick learners.

Mrs Savage: What are the long-term consequences of uncontrolled blood sugar levels?

Doctor: The bad news is that once you get diabetes you have it for good and it can cause a lot of complications. The good news is that you can control it and with good control you can reduce the chances of having complications.

It generally takes several years (usually about 10 years) for the long-term complications of diabetes to evolve, though the changes start within the first 4 years. Maintaining a good blood sugar level reduces the risk of these complications. Abnormal levels could affect Paul's physical growth. Diabetes can affect the blood vessels and the nerves over a period of several years.

Small blood vessels in the retina, the layer of tissue at the back of the eye that is responsible for vision, may be affected, causing a condition called retinopathy. If this is left untreated it can lead to loss of sight. We will be checking Paul's eyes at least once a year. We have a screening service in this hospital, so please don't worry. The other thing we would look for would be a cataract when the lens of the eye becomes opaque.

The small vessels of the kidneys can also be affected, causing serious kidney problems that could eventually need dialysis. Diabetes can also affect the nerve endings causing problems over a period of several years. Paul is also more susceptible to pick up infections because diabetes compromises the body's defence mechanisms.

As Paul gets older he could be more at risk of developing high cholesterol, heart problems, and skin problems. In short, diabetes quickens the pace of all the problems of old age, but by keeping good control of the blood sugar levels it is possible to reduce the risk of having these long-term complications.

Mrs Savage: What about his diet?

Doctor: It is crucial that Paul has a balanced diet and he has already seen our dietitian. He is an intelligent boy and a fast learner. He has already grasped the basic principles of his diet from Mrs Shaw. He understands that he should have a good diet with less fat and more fibre. Mrs Shaw will go through the list of things that Paul can and cannot have in detail with you. She will also give you a booklet about diet in diabetes. Don't worry. Paul will learn it quick enough.

Here is an information leaflet about diabetes. It explains all the issues that I have discussed with you today. I would suggest that you join the British Diabetic Association (or BDA). The leaflet gives you the addresses and various contact phone numbers. You can also join the local branch of the BDA and the local self-help group if you would like to be able to meet other people in the same situation as yourself. The BDA also organizes holiday camps and educational trips and Paul could join the ones he likes.

Mrs Savage: Will diabetes affect Paul's overall development?

Doctor: Most children with diabetes grow up to be normal adults. It is certainly possible for Paul to achieve his full potential. He can go to school, play, and have fun like any other kid of his age. Of course, the only difference from other kids is that he needs insulin injections. You probably don't know this, but Steve Redgrave, who got his fifth Olympic gold medal in 2000, is an insulin-dependent diabetic. I can assure you that you will soon meet many other people with diabetes who lead active and fulfilling lives.

Mrs Savage: What about my other two sons? Are they at risk of having diabetes as well?

Doctor: The risk of Paul's brothers developing diabetes is about 1 in 20. However, at the moment it is not possible to predict accurately whether or not they will develop diabetes. Is there anything else you would like to ask me?

Mrs Savage: No, thank you, doctor.

Doctor: OK, Mrs Savage. I realize that this is a lot to take in, though I expect it is not all new to you as your father had diabetes. Please feel free to ask any other questions when I next see you and I will go over this information again. It is difficult to absorb it all in one session. I will see you again before Paul goes home.

Mr Sharp, a 23-year-old man, has been diagnosed with epilepsy. He is being discharged from hospital. You are the SHO on the firm. It is important that you see him before he goes home. What advice would you give him?

The diagnosis of epilepsy causes a lot of distress and anxiety to patients and their relatives. It is always useful to take the time to explain what epilepsy means. People often have a very old-fashioned view about epilepsy and mistakenly think that epileptic patients have defective or subnormal brains. Patients usually like to know about:

- The cause of the epilepsy
- Treatment
- Side effects of the drugs
- How this might affect their social life
- Implications for work and driving
- What they can do to help themselves
- Whether it is genetic

Doctor: Good afternoon, Mr Sharp. I am delighted to tell you that you can go home today. However, I must have a chat with you about your condition, what it all means, and how it is going to affect you.

Mr Sharp: Thanks, I'd like to ask a few questions.

Doctor: Well, as you know, you were admitted to the hospital last week with fits. This is the second time that you have had them, which means that you have a tendency to recurring epileptic seizures. We must try and prevent these from happening and that is why we have started you on regular treatment.

We have done several blood investigations, a tracing of the electrical activity of the brain and a CT scan of the brain. There is definitely no evidence of a brain tumour or of any other structural abnormality. I am very happy to reassure you about that.

Mr Sharp: That is good news that the brain scan didn't show anything sinister. But what is the cause of the epilepsy and why did I get it?

Doctor: Let me explain what happens. The brain cells communicate with each other by means of electric currents, but these do not spread to the entire brain and are kept in check by these cells. An unchecked single electric discharge affecting the whole brain produces an epileptic seizure. Although the cause of epilepsy is not entirely known, a previous brain injury and occasionally some structural abnormalities in the brain can cause such seizures. In your situation, as you know, we have not found any cause and often we don't. We call this form of epilepsy 'idiopathic' which means 'the one where no cause is known'.

Mr Sharp: Is it genetic? Is my son likely to get it?

Doctor: I quite understand your anxiety. We know that genetic factors can influence the development of epilepsy, but it is difficult to assess the risk in a particular case accurately. About 2% of the population have had two or more seizures. This 1 in 50 risk becomes 1 in 3 for first-degree relatives of an epileptic patient.

Mr Sharp: What can I do to prevent another attack?

Doctor: You can actually do a lot of things to help yourself. First of all, try to relax, and don't get too anxious about having another attack. Secondly, it is very important that you take your medications regularly. Carbamazepine, the drug that you are on, is very effective in controlling fits. Thirdly, there are some well-known precipitating factors such as alcoholic binges and flickering lights and you should try to avoid these.

We may have to check the blood levels of carbamazepine in a few weeks, just to make sure that the blood level is within acceptable and effective limits.

Mr Sharp: Does this drug have any side-effects?

Doctor: Carbamazepine is fairly well tolerated by most patients. However, it does have some side-effects that you need to know about. It can cause unsteadiness and dizziness. Some patients have also reported double vision. It can give you tummy upsets. Very occasionally it can affect the liver, causing jaundice, and the bone marrow, causing infections. If you experience any of these symptoms you should contact us immediately. I am giving you a long list but that does not mean that you will get all of these, just that it is a good idea to be aware of them. Carbamazepine also interacts with some other drugs, so if another doctor, who does not know what medication you are on, prescribes something for you then you should mention it to him.

Mr Sharp: Is there anything that I should *not* be doing? What about sex?

Doctor: You must take some simple, commonsense precautions so that you do not place yourself in a situation where a fit will expose you to danger. Avoid swimming and cycling alone. Take a shallow bath, and only if someone else is at home. Do not lock the bathroom door. Avoid working with heavy moving machinery. You should inform the DVLA as you are not allowed to drive until you have been fit-free for at least 2 years or have had fits only at night for 3 years. You will never be able to drive a public service vehicle — that's the law I'm afraid. You can return to normal sexual activity straightaway.

Mr Sharp: What about alcohol? And can I play football?

Doctor: Alcohol consumption in moderation is fine but, as I said, you must avoid binges. You can play football and there is no problem with that. However, there are certain occupations you will not be allowed to take up — essentially those in which you pose any risk to yourself or someone else, such as childminding or tree surgery, or those that involve climbing, such as a steeplejack or a window cleaner.

You should carry an epilepsy card with you all the time. You could also join the local epilepsy support group. There are a number of leaflets here which contain useful information about a lot of things. Please take a copy of each. You will find the Internet addresses on them as well.

I have made an appointment to see you in the clinic in 2 months but do not hesitate to contact us immediately if you have any new problems. Is there anything else that you would like to ask me?

Mr Sharp: Should I tell other people?

Doctor: Unfortunately, people with epilepsy do sometimes encounter prejudice, especially when seeking employment. This prejudice is based on the common misconceptions that epilepsy is invariably associated with mental retardation and neurological disease and that epileptics are in some way 'freaks'. These old beliefs are gradually changing, albeit very slowly.

On balance, it is probably best to tell people you meet frequently so that you can educate them about the condition, and advise them what to do if a seizure occurs when you are with them. I'm sure that your friends will appreciate your showing confidence in them in this way. Is there anything else you would like to ask me?

Mr Sharp: No, thank you.

Doctor: Take care. I'll be seeing you in 8 weeks.

Jamie, an 8-month-old boy, is being discharged from the hospital after an episode of febrile convulsions. You are the paediatric SHO. Talk to his anxious mother.

Seeing one's child have a fit is a distressing experience. Parents are very worried and will be anxious to ask questions about:

- The cause of febrile convulsions
- The risk of epilepsy in the future
- The risk of brain damage
- How to prevent it from happening again
- What to do if it happens again

Doctor: Good afternoon, Mrs Armitage. I am delighted to let you know that Jamie can be discharged from the hospital today. I would like to talk to you first about his recent illness — I'm sure that you have some questions you would like to ask.

Mrs Armitage: Thank you for seeing me, doctor. Yes, I am still confused about what a febrile convulsion is and how it comes about. Could you explain it to me again?

Doctor: Certainly. As you know, Jamie had a sore throat which gave him a high fever. In fact his temperature was 40°C. High temperatures in some babies can cause an abnormal electrical activity in the brain and it is this that produces the fit. Fits due to high fevers are called 'febrile convulsions'. Although we are not entirely sure why some babies have fits with fever and others don't, febrile convulsions are not uncommon in babies.

Mrs Armitage: Can it cause brain damage? Is Jamie at risk?

Doctor: I can understand your anxiety but you need not worry. As you know, Jamie had a fit lasting for about 2 to 3 minutes. This is unlikely to have caused any brain damage. In general, the longer the fits last the higher the risk of brain damage. Anyway, I have examined him again today and I found no evidence of any brain damage.

Mrs Armitage: Will Jamie develop epilepsy in the future?

Doctor: That is a very difficult question to answer. I must stress first of all that a febrile convulsion, even though it may recur, is *not* epilepsy. We do know, however, that babies who have had febrile convulsions do have a higher risk of developing epilepsy in later life, although estimating that risk for one particular baby is extremely difficult.

Mrs Armitage: Do you think he will get these fits again — or have them all his life?

Doctor: Jamie is certainly at risk of having febrile convulsions again if he has another high temperature. However, you will be relieved to know that most children outgrow the tendency to have these fits as they grow older, usually by the age of 3 years.

Mrs Armitage: What should I do if he has a fit with a high fever at home?

Doctor: Well, the first thing to consider is how to *prevent* a fit in the first place. If you suspect that Jamie has an infection and is feverish you must check his temperature. You can do this by placing a thermometer strip on his forehead — you can buy these quite cheaply from a chemist. If the temperature is 38°C or higher, put Jamie on a bed and undress him. Get two facecloths and a bucket of tepid water. Make sure that the water is not too cold. Dip both the cloths in water and wring them out so they don't drip. Put one cloth on his forehead and the other on one of his arms. Remove the first cloth, rinse it and wring it out and place it on the other arm. You can cool down the forehead, armpits, arms, soles, groins and legs by going round them with the cloths. This is a good way of reducing the baby's temperature and preventing the possibility of a fit.

Also, give him a teaspoon of paediatric paracetamol syrup straightaway. This will also help to bring down his temperature. Have some rectal diazepam handy, the drug that has been prescribed for you to take home, just in case, and call your GP because if Jamie has an infection it will need to be treated.

If you think Jamie *is* having a fit don't panic. Put him in the recovery position — either on his right or his left side, not on his back — so that his airway remains open. Make sure that there is nothing hard nearby which he could hurt himself against. Put one diazepam suppository into his back passage and get him to Casualty immediately.

All this is explained in this leaflet. Please take it home and have a good look at it. Do you have any other questions?

Mrs Armitage: Will Jamie develop normally?

Doctor: Yes, Mrs Armitage, most babies who have had febrile convulsions develop into normal, healthy, active children. Don't worry. I have made an appointment to see Jamie in the clinic in 6 weeks. If there are any problems get in touch with your GP surgery. I will be writing to them about Jamie.

Mrs Deacon, a 56-year-old lady, was told when she was an inpatient in the hospital that she has the irritable bowel syndrome. You are the medical SHO in the clinic and she asks you for an explanation of what this is and whether there is anything special that she should be doing.

The irritable bowel syndrome is a common condition. Psychological stress often triggers attacks. Your patient is likely to ask you a lot of questions but her main concerns will probably be:

- What is the irritable bowel syndrome and what causes it?
- Is there any treatment?
- Is there anything she can do to stop it from flaring up?
- Can it cause cancer of the bowel?

Doctor: Good morning, Mrs Deacon. Come in and take a seat. How are you today?

Mrs Deacon: I'm fine, doctor. I wonder if you would explain to me exactly, what this 'irritable syndrome' means. Why my bowels are so irritable?

Doctor: Yes, certainly. As you know, you were admitted with abdominal pain and diarrhoea. You have had bouts of diarrhoea, abdominal pain, and constipation for some time. We did some blood tests, stool tests, and a sigmoidoscopy to make sure that there was nothing seriously wrong with your bowel. Based on your symptoms and their long history, we came to the conclusion that you have a very sensitive and nervous gut, and this state — it is not really a *disease* — is called the irritable bowel syndrome, or IBS for short. We certainly did not find anything nasty in the bowel. Small and hard faeces cause the bowel muscle to contract harder and this contraction is felt in the tummy like a cramp. Abdominal pain, a bloated sensation, diarrhoea, and constipation are the usual symptoms of IBS.

Mrs Deacon: Yes, they mentioned this. I have heard of IBS before. Can you explain what causes it, doctor?

Doctor: Yes, of course. It is a very common problem and affects a lot of people. It usually occurs about the time of middle age, when you are still in an active period of your life. It is rare in children but can happen in them as well. What seems to happen is that some people's anxious disposition manifests itself through their gut which becomes irritable and goes into spasms. These cause pains, constipation, and diarrhoea. Food is normally moved along the bowel by the contractions of the muscles in the bowel wall. Sometimes these contractions get out of their normal rhythm, causing the muscles to go into spasm, and this gives rise to the tummy pains. Some patients are also abnormally sensitive to distension of the bowel, though it does not have to be very distended to cause problems. This is called 'heightened visceral perception' and it causes a sensation of being bloated. Unfortunately this also increases the contractility of the muscle and gives rise to even more tummy pain. We are not entirely sure why this happens.

Mrs Deacon: What can be done to control these pains, doctor?

Doctor: You can do a lot to help yourself. The most important thing is to try to reduce any stress and anxiety in your life. There is evidence to suggest that stress can bring on the symptoms. I know that it can be very difficult to reduce stress if there are family or financial problems, but worrying about them is only going to make things worse. Relaxation exercises can be helpful to some extent. I happen to have a video and an audiotape on relaxation that I could lend you if you would like to try them.

Watch what you eat. A good diet for IBS is one that is high in fibre and low in fat and sugar. I will see that you get an information sheet on this kind of diet. Fibre is the most important thing and high-fibre foods include bran, peas and pods, green vegetables, and wholemeal bread. That said, unfortunately some patients find that their bowels become *more* irritable on high-fibre diets. Our dietitian will help you to find the right combination of things to eat. Avoid salt, convenience foods, bacon, sausages, crisps, peanuts, and Marmite. If any other foods seem to make your bowels worse then try to avoid them too.

You may just have to accept this condition as an expression of your 'bowel personality' in a way and learn to live with your symptoms. I will give you something to take if your pains become troublesome but it would be preferable if you could manage to ignore these pains and the irregularity of your bowels. We can also increase your fibre intake by giving you some sachets of fibre to take with water twice a day. This would help keep your bowels regular.

Mrs Deacon, it is important to remember that you must be patient. The symptoms caused by IBS can take some time to settle as you make adjustments in your lifestyle and diet. You may find that you start to have long, trouble-free periods and that eventually the condition will settle down.

Mrs Deacon: Will it cause any long-term problems? Can it go on to develop into bowel cancer, for example?

Doctor: IBS does not predispose to cancer of the bowel. It also does not cause chronic inflammatory bowel disease or colitis.

Mrs Deacon: Will it go away completely?

Doctor: We can certainly control the symptoms with medication if they become troublesome. As I said, you should realize that the irritable bowel syndrome is a state and not a disease, and as such it cannot be cured completely. However, a lot can be done along the lines I have suggested to keep it under control and it will gradually settle down. If you need further information about IBS you can contact the IBS Network in London. Here is an information leaflet about it which you might find useful. Is there anything else you would like to ask me?

Mrs Deacon: No, thank you.

Doctor: Come back and see me if you have any new problems or if the symptoms get out of control.

Mrs Scott, a 52-year-old lady, has symptoms of the menopause. You are the SHO in the endocrine clinic. Talk to her about her problems and about the advantages and disadvantages of hormone replacement therapy.

Although the menopause is a natural phenomenon and most women of this patient's age could be expected to know quite a lot about it, there are some who do not fully understand all its manifestations. Be sure to explain the physiological processes that underlie the symptoms and the treatment with some sensitivity. After highlighting both the benefits and the drawbacks of hormone replacement therapy, encourage her to decide herself if she considers that the advantages outweigh the potential risks.

Mrs Scott: Doctor, I have been having hot flushes and sweating. My periods have also stopped being regular and I don't lose much blood. Some of my friends tell me that I am going through 'the change'. Are they right?

Doctor: Yes, it would seem so, Mrs Scott. Irregular periods, sometimes with hot flushes, precede the menopause, or the change. This happens in most women between the ages of 45 and 55 years, although in some women it can happen sooner or later than this. Around this age the ovaries become less active and the level of the female hormone, oestrogen, falls. Oestrogen deficiency causes hot flushes, sweating, dryness of the skin, and dryness of the vagina which is sometimes associated with dyspareunia, or pain during sexual intercourse. It also causes a decrease in the size of the breasts, and urinary frequency and urgency. Many women also experience psychological symptoms such as mood changes and a lack of interest in sex. I'm afraid this is a long list but mercifully not everyone gets all the symptoms.

Mrs Scott: I have some of these symptoms. Is there anything you can give me for them?

Doctor: Before I come to the treatment let me tell you something about the long-term effects of oestrogen deficiency. This is important because the symptoms themselves are not permanent and are often tolerable. They may not need any treatment and you must really think more about the *long-term* benefits and risks of any treatment. Before the menopause, women do not get as many heart attacks as men do at a comparable age, but they start catching up with men as their ovaries get tired and stop producing female hormones. Low oestrogen also causes thinning of the bones, or osteoporosis, which causes bone fractures in many women after the menopause.

Supplying these hormones to women after the menopause, when the ovaries no longer produce them themselves is called 'hormone replacement therapy', or HRT for short. HRT usually relieves most menopausal symptoms and prevents osteoporosis. If given for 10 years from the menopause, HRT reduces strokes and halves the risk of fractures due to thinning of the bones as it does the risk of heart attacks. A fringe benefit seems to be that the incidence of Alzheimer's disease is lower in women on HRT, and the onset of the disease is delayed compared with women who are not on long-term treatment.

Unfortunately, there is a debit side too. HRT may cause nausea, an increase in appetite with weight gain, breast swelling and tenderness, and vaginal discharge. The risk of forming clots in the veins is about two to four times higher in women on HRT. Women taking HRT for longer than 10 years have a slightly increased risk of developing breast cancer, but this needs to be confirmed by further long-term studies. Withdrawal bleeding due to the treatment itself is sometimes very troublesome in women taking both progestogen and oestrogen. I will tell you more about the different forms of HRT if you decide to go ahead with it.

Mrs Scott: Do I have any alternative?

Doctor: Well, it is important to understand what is going on in your body in the menopause, and that it is a natural process that all women go through as they get older. You may be interested to know that men have the menopause too! If you understand what is happening it will be easier to accept the menopause and its symptoms, particularly if they are not too troublesome.

Smoking decreases oestrogen levels in the blood and if you are a smoker you should give it up. A healthy diet, rich in calcium, may help prevent osteoporosis. Foods that are high in calcium include milk and cheese, broccoli, baked beans, oranges, salmon, and sardines. If you would like some information about diet you could speak to a dietitian, or look through one of the many books on diets in your local library. Take regular exercise. This will strengthen your bones and help your heart as well. Try to spend time out-of-doors. This is important because your skin requires sunlight to produce a chemical called vitamin D that increases the calcium level in your body. Make sure, though, that you use sunscreen creams to avoid sunburn. Lastly, a stress-free lifestyle and a supportive partner can make all the difference.

Apart from HRT there are other medications available, such as clonidine for hot flushes. Antidepressants help some patients, and drugs such as raloxifene and bisphosphonates can be used to control postmenopausal osteoporosis.

There are also many alternative treatments available. Aromatherapy can help you to relax. Acupuncture, homeopathy and herbal remedies are thought to be useful and although there is no definite evidence to show that they are beneficial, they do not appear to be harmful either. Soya flour contains oestrogenic compounds but its benefits have not been convincing.

Starting HRT has significant implications and you will have to consider the pros and cons carefully before deciding to start treatment. Here is an information sheet explaining everything in detail. Have a think about it and get back to me over the next few days. Now, is there anything else you would like to ask me?

Mrs Scott: No doctor, not at the moment. But I might take you up on your offer and ask you some more questions once I have had time to think it all over. Thank you.

Mr Ramsay, a 62-year-old man, is being discharged after recovering from a myocardial infarction. You are the SHO on the medical firm. Give him some advice about what he can and cannot do.

To make best use of this opportunity to counsel your patient you should assess his level of knowledge about his condition and identify his main concerns. You should be able to find out how much he knows from the initial pleasantries. The anxieties of a patient who is recovering from a myocardial infarction will be about:

■ Their heart — if it has been badly damaged; how long it will take to recover; if there will be any permanent damage
■ Life after a heart attack — any changes that will have to be made
■ The likelihood of further attacks

Although you might like to emphasize straightaway the importance of such things as regular exercise and medication, you should encourage him first to ask questions so that you can address his specific concerns. He should know by now what a heart attack means but if no one has explained, or he is hazy about it, you should explain it in simple terms. Most major hospitals have a Cardiac Rehabilitation Programme and someone may have approached him already — if not, you should reassure him that you will arrange this for him.

Doctor: Good morning, Mr Ramsay. How are you this morning?

Mr Ramsay: Fine, thank you.

Doctor: I know that you are being discharged today. You must be looking forward to going home.

Mr Ramsay: Yes, very much so.

Doctor: There are a few things I need to explain before you go home. You know you have had a heart attack — do you know what that means? (*Give him time to explain in his own way and add any pieces of information as you go along. We shall assume here that he needs a full explanation.*)

Well, the heart is a muscular pump and when it contracts it sends blood containing oxygen and nutrients to all parts of the body. The heart needs a blood supply of its own to provide fuel for it to work. This is done through three fuel pipes, or blood vessels, called the coronary arteries. The harder the heart has to work, for example when you exercise or are excited, the more fuel it needs which is no problem if the blood vessels are normal. In coronary artery disease there is patchy furring up of the inside of the blood vessels causing narrowing. This process is known as 'atheroma'. A patch of atheroma may develop a crack and a clot, or thrombosis, can build up over this and block the artery. The heart muscle that was relying on this blocked artery is starved of blood and becomes damaged after half an hour or so. A myocardial infarction or heart attack is what we call this damage.

The most important thing to remember is that you have recovered from this attack and your heart should serve you as well in the future as it did in the past. (*Pause.*) The heart is a strong organ and has remarkable powers of recovery. The healing process will already have started and in about 6 weeks the scar on your heart muscle will have completely healed. (*This is assuming that he has made an uneventful recovery. At any rate, a little optimism is well placed in such cases.*)

You may feel tired or listless, anxious and irritable, or depressed, for a week or so at home. All that is normal and most people experience such a reaction. You will need both rest and exercise — the trick is to get the balance right. Have 7 to 8 hours of sleep at night and rest in the afternoon whenever you feel like it. After a few days of rest at home gentle, but gradually increasing, exercise will help you to get fitter. One of the physiotherapists may have already come to see you but, if not, I will arrange it and they will discuss exercise with you.

There is an active Cardiac Rehabilitation Programme in this hospital and I will arrange for someone from that team to speak with you. They have leaflets which explain what you can and cannot do. They also have some literature from the British Heart Foundation which gives useful information. The main thing is to increase your exercise gradually, a bit more each day, and rest when you feel tired or if you have chest pain.

Basically, at home you should be doing similar activities to those you have been doing in hospital and then gradually increase them. Do not compare yourself with other people and do not eat immediately before exercise. By the end of 6 weeks after discharge you should be taking regular daily exercise and should even be more active than you were before your heart attack. Avoid pushing or pulling heavy weights — remember, the accent is on activity and getting fitter to enjoy an active life.

The medication that you are taking home with you includes aspirin, which thins the blood and prevents a clot from forming; atenolol, which slows down the heart; simvastatin, which will keep your blood cholesterol level below 4–8 mmol/L; and an ACE inhibitor, which stops the heart from becoming weak. It is important that you take these medications regularly. It will help you to remember when to take them if you take them when you are doing something else that you do regularly, such as brushing your teeth. You mustn't stop any medicines without consulting your doctor — that can be dangerous. Is there anything more you would like to know about your medication?

Mr Ramsay: No, but what about other things? For example, when can I go back to work?

Doctor: After about 8 weeks many people are fit enough to return to work, depending on the nature of their work. You should consult your GP first. In general, it is often advisable to start back to work, including any household chores, on a part-time basis for the first few weeks until you get used to the routine of working again. There are certain jobs that people may not be able to return to after they have had a heart attack, however, such as driving trains, heavy goods vehicles, or public service vehicles. You should discuss going back to work with your GP.

Mr Ramsay: I presume I may have more of these attacks?

Doctor: You may never have another heart attack but it is impossible to say with confidence whether or not or when you will have another attack. However, you can do a lot to prevent one by trying to reduce the various risk factors, such as high blood pressure, smoking, stress, and your cholesterol level. Your blood pressure will have been checked here, but you should have it checked again during your recovery programme. Similarly, you will need to have your cholesterol level checked. You should take a low-fat, high-fibre diet. I can give you some leaflets from our Dietetic Department. If you are a smoker you must give it up completely — it is never too late to give up. You should also try to avoid breathing in other people's smoke.

Alcohol in moderation, up to about 21 units a week, is not harmful to your coronary arteries, but heavy drinking can weaken the heart muscle and increase your weight. Stress is harmful if it gets out of control. Avoid overwork and the stress of working to deadlines, and arguments. Try to plan your workload, perhaps delegate some work; take up a new hobby; and exercise more.

You are probably wondering about driving and about sex. (*Pause.*) The current regulations suggest that you cannot drive for a month; leave it longer if you feel that your reflexes are not back to their usual level. You should not travel by air for at least 6 weeks after your heart attack.

Your heart will be able to cope with the stresses of sex but it will take 2 to 4 weeks of your exercise programme before you are fit enough. The effect on the heart of having intercourse is comparable to running up three flights of stairs. Remember though that your partner will still need you to show affection in other ways.

Now, is there anything that I haven't discussed or anything that you would like to bring up? Please feel free to ask anything — if I don't know the answer then I will find someone who does.

Mr Ramsay: No, there isn't anything else. Thank you, doctor.

Mrs Marks, a 20-year-old lady, was admitted to hospital with severe headache of sudden onset. She has been found to have migraine. You are the neurology SHO. Explain to her what migraine means. Also explain to her what the 'aura' or warning signs of migraine are, and how to recognize and handle an attack of migraine at home.

Migraine is a common condition that can have significant physical and social implications for many patients. Patients usually ask:

- What causes migraine?
- What treatment is available?
- How can I prevent an attack of migraine?
- What should I do during an attack?
- Is it inherited?

Doctor: Hello, Mrs Marks. How are you today?

Mrs Marks: I am fine, doctor. Do you have the results of the tests I had?

Doctor: As you know, you came into hospital with a severe headache. We did several tests and I am glad to say that all these tests have come back as normal. We think that your headache was due to migraine. There is no evidence of anything more serious. I expect that you have been concerned that you might have a brain tumour or something like that.

Mrs Marks: Yes, I was a bit worried about that. I am relieved that there is nothing serious. What exactly is migraine? I have heard the name but don't know what it means. My headaches were really very severe.

Doctor: Well, to put it in simple terms, migraine is a form of headache that occurs when one or more of the branches of a big blood vessel called the carotid artery that supply your scalp dilates abnormally. The exact mechanism is not known but certain chemicals, such as serotonin, have been blamed. There are several types of headache caused by a disturbance of blood vessels and migraine is one of these. Migraine itself has various types, including classic migraine, common migraine, migraine equivalent, and complicated migraine. It is quite a common condition and affects about 1 in 10 of the population, the vast majority of them being women.

Mrs Marks: Will the headaches come back again?

Doctor: Yes, I'm afraid it is a recurring condition. You may only get an attack every 6 or 9 months if you are lucky, but some people have more frequent attacks, as often as once a month or more. The most important part of managing migraine is *prevention*. First of all, we try to identify trigger factors — any particular situations or activity, or anything you eat or drink that brings on an attack. Avoiding the trigger factors is one way of preventing migrainous headaches.

Mrs Marks: How do I identify the trigger factors? Are there any common ones that I need to know about?

Doctor: One way of identifying trigger factors is to keep a diary in which you record the date and the time of any headaches, making a note of what you had been doing or eating during the previous 24 hours. This can help you to find out your trigger factors. Missing meals, as well as eating things that do not suit you, can bring on migraine. In some patients, alcohol, cheese, chocolate, tea and coffee, or fried foods can trigger attacks of migraine. If you suspect that certain foods or drinks may bring on an attack, record when you eat or drink these things and see if the headaches start soon afterwards. If they do, then try to avoid that particular food for 4 weeks. If the headaches stop you may have found the answer.

Stress, either emotional or physical, can cause migraines. Also avoid extremes of temperature and too much sunbathing. Be particularly careful with bright dazzling lights such as the ones used at discos. Avoid looking at the television when the picture is flickering. You may have to avoid driving at night as the headlights of oncoming vehicles can cause attacks. Noise, driving a car or riding a bicycle can make your headache worse. Sometimes, menstrual periods can bring on an attack.

Mrs Marks: Can I take any tablets to prevent these attacks from happening?

Doctor: Yes, there are several drugs available to prevent attacks. If you are getting frequent attacks of migraine, once or twice a month, we would think about prescribing something for you. It usually takes at least 2 weeks for the drug to start to work. About 60% to 75% of patients seem to benefit from such treatment.

Mrs Marks: You told me that there are various types of migraine. Which one do I have?

Doctor: You had what I call a 'full house', an aura with visual disturbance, a one-sided headache, and nausea. These are the features of classic migraine.

Mrs Marks: Would you explain the aura in a bit more detail, please?

Doctor: OK. Before the headache starts you may get a warning which is called an 'aura', and you may experience some unusual sensations. These sensations are usually visual and may consist of flashing or zigzagging lights, dimness of vision, or a sensation of looking through water. Very occasionally, people may even experience temporary blindness. Rarely, you may be feeling perfectly well but suddenly become conscious of a bright spot on one side of your vision. This may slowly get bigger and spread, becoming darker in the centre. Sometimes you may get a tingling feeling or numbness in one side of the face or around the lips, or have pins and needles down one side of your body. An aura may also occur in the form of weakness of one of your arms or legs. Uncommon warning symptoms include difficulty in speaking and mental confusion.

These symptoms can be frightening but fortunately do not last long. It is important that you are able to recognize these symptoms as they may herald an attack of headache, giving you an early warning, and enabling you to deal with the attack more effectively.

Mrs Marks: What should I do if I have an attack of migraine at home?

Doctor: If you have recognized the symptoms of an aura and you feel that a headache is impending, the first thing to do is not to panic. Try to relax. If the headache strikes suddenly, take two paracetamol tablets and go to bed in a dark room for an hour or two. Just lie flat, relax, and gently massage your forehead. Cold compresses can be very soothing. If your headaches are associated with vomiting you should take a tablet that I will give you to prevent that. Rebreathing into a paper bag may sometimes stop an attack. If the headache is not responding or gets worse you should contact your GP or come to hospital. You should also consider doing that if your headache seems unusual or is of sudden onset.

Mrs Marks: Is it inherited? Will I pass it on to my children? No one else in my family has had migraine.

Doctor: There is what we call a 'hereditary predisposition' but at the present time it is very difficult to quantify that risk.

Mrs Marks: Can I go on the 'pill'? Is it safe?

Doctor: Well, we know that oral contraceptive pills can make migraine worse in about a third of patients. Therefore, if you go on the 'pill' you should monitor your attacks carefully: if the headaches get worse or if you get any new neurological symptoms you should stop taking it and see your GP. Is there anything else you would like to ask me?

Mrs Marks: No, thank you.

Doctor: Here are some pamphlets on migraine. They give you information about migraine, self-help groups, and some useful websites. You may find them helpful.

Take care, Mrs Marks. Do not hesitate to contact your GP if you have any new problems. We will not need to see you in clinic unless there are difficulties that your GP would like further advice about.

Miss Stewart, a 24-year-old lady, has been diagnosed with multiple sclerosis. You are the neurology SHO and she has come to see you in the clinic. Your task is to explain the diagnosis and the possible course of her disease.

The diagnosis of multiple sclerosis will have come as a shock to the patient and, understandably, it causes a lot of anxiety. In the past, unless a patient asked for the exact diagnosis, many doctors would use some euphemism to explain the condition, such as 'inflammatory spots in the brain'. In these days of greater patient involvement and better communication, doctors are encouraged to give the exact diagnosis and more information to patients. Nonetheless, receiving such news is as frightening now as it was in the past, and giving the patient an explanation of the condition before delivering the diagnosis may dilute its shocking impact. Be understanding and patient when you answer her questions, which will probably include:

- What causes multiple sclerosis?
- What are the treatment options?
- How is this going to affect me in the future?
- Is it inherited?

Doctor: Good morning, Miss Stewart.

Miss Stewart: Good morning, doctor. This is my partner, John. I hope you don't mind if he joins me during this consultation.

Doctor: Of course not. Nice to meet you, John. Well, Miss Stewart, you have been in hospital for over a week now and all your symptoms of blurred vision and numbness of the hands have gone. How are you feeling now?

Miss Stewart: Fine. All these problems have disappeared now. I don't have any numbness of my fingers and my vision is back to normal. As you know, though, I had similar symptoms a few months ago, when they disappeared a day or so later. Do you have the results of all the tests that I have had during the last few days?

Doctor: Yes, certainly. You had some blood tests, an MRI scan of the brain, and some neurophysiological studies which were testing how the messages from your eyes are received by your brain. These tests suggest that your symptoms were due to patchy damage to the sheaths that insulate your nerves. This is affecting more than one nerve and that is why you have been getting symptoms in several parts of the body. Do you have any idea yourself what this condition might be?

Miss Stewart: No, doctor, I don't.

Doctor: Let me explain what happens. A material called myelin forms sheaths around the nerves in your body, just like the rubber sheaths used to coat electric wires for insulation. These myelin sheaths insulate the conduction of electric nerve impulses along your nerves. Damage to them is called 'demyelination', which means that the sheaths have been denuded in some places. These bare patches interfere with the smooth conduction of nerve impulses and cause the symptoms that you have had. The condition is therefore described as a 'demyelinating' disease (*pause*); because the denuding process affects many nerves it is more commonly referred to as 'multiple sclerosis'. (*Pause.*) You have probably heard of this before.

Miss Stewart: I have heard of it but I don't know much about it except that it is a dreadful disease.

Doctor: Well, not necessarily and not in every case. I can't pretend that it is pleasant or that its outcome is rosy, but it takes different forms. You may get further episodes like the ones you had, or you may get some other symptoms. They usually resolve, as they did in your case, but sometimes you can be left with some degree of weakness. It all depends on how much damage has occurred in the nervous system. At one extreme, there are some patients who have a benign form of the disease with no significant disability for many years; at the opposite extreme are the 10% to 15% of patients who have progressive symptoms from the outset, with no relapses and remissions. It looks as if you are among those who have relapses and remissions of the disease that may go on for many years.

Miss Stewart: What causes this damage?

Doctor: The cause of multiple sclerosis is not entirely known. There is some evidence to suggest that problems with the immune system, viral infections, and genetic factors may each play some role in the cause of this disease. However, it is true to say that we do not have all the answers yet.

Miss Stewart: Is there any treatment for multiple sclerosis?

Doctor: Many forms of treatment have been tried, but unfortunately without much effect on the eventual outcome. Some drugs such as steroids and ACTH can be given to reduce the severity of a relapse. Beta interferon may reduce the rate of relapse and you would qualify for this treatment as you have already had two relapses in less than a year. My boss, Professor Pinkerton, has a special interest in this disease and he is participating in a large trial that is due to start soon. He will consider whether or not you might benefit from treatment with Beta interferon and keep your name on his books so that if there are any other new advances you can be considered for them too.

Miss Stewart: Is there anything I could do to prevent these symptoms from happening again?

Doctor: Yes, there are some rather general measures. Have a balanced diet, avoid exertion, and try to relax. Try to avoid stressful situations.

Miss Stewart: What about alcohol and smoking?

Doctor: There seems to be no evidence that alcohol and smoking aggravate multiple sclerosis. However, it is always advisable to drink only in moderation and, of course, it is better not to smoke if you want to maintain a healthy lifestyle.

Miss Stewart: What about the future? Will I end up in a wheelchair?

Doctor: I fully understand your anxiety. As I said before it is very hard to predict how this condition is going to behave in an individual case. Studies have shown that nearly half of all the patients studied were in full-time work in the first 5 years following diagnosis and that the majority were capable of useful work. Someone like you with purely visual and sensory symptoms has a much better outlook in the long term. Patients with frequent, prolonged relapses, with incomplete recovery, and those with progressive disease have a poor prognosis. For patients who are unlucky and develop physical disability, however, there is a lot of help and many support services available. Most patients lead a productive life.

Miss Stewart: How about sex or pregnancy?

Doctor: Multiple sclerosis does not reduce your fertility so you would be able to have children. There is no increased risk of miscarriage, no specific complications in labour, and no problem with breastfeeding. During pregnancy you might find that the frequency of attacks may reduce, though some patients find that they have more relapses during the first 3 months after pregnancy. On the whole, pregnancy does not particularly affect the course of the disease.

Miss Stewart: Is it inherited? Would any children I might have be at risk?

Doctor: There is a genetic susceptibility but the risk is very small. Is there anything else you would like to ask me, or do you want to ask anything, John?

Miss Stewart: No, thank you.

John: No, I think you have covered everything.

Doctor: Here is an information sheet on multiple sclerosis. It gives you a list of Internet sites and the telephone number of the local branch of the Multiple Sclerosis Society, which you could join if you think that would be helpful. Your next appointment is in 6 weeks when you will see Professor Pinkerton. You can discuss all this with him then a bit more fully, but you can always contact me earlier if you have any problems.

Tim, a 9-month-old baby, has a nappy rash. His mother, Mrs North, is very worried. You are the paediatric SHO and your task is to reassure her, explain the diagnosis to her, and give her any relevant information.

Most people have heard of nappy rash, and many will recognize it quite easily, but it can still be a very unpleasant and unsettling sight. Tim's mother will need to have answers to these questions:

- What is nappy rash and what causes it?
- How is it treated?
- How can it be prevented?

Doctor: Mrs North, please do take a chair. Let's have a brief chat about Tim's rash. You have probably heard someone call it a 'nappy rash'.

Mrs North: Yes, doctor, but what *is* nappy rash and what causes it?

Doctor: Nappy rash is an area of red, angry-looking spots that affects the part of the bottom covered by the nappy. It can be very sore and causes the baby a lot of discomfort. It is a very common condition and affects up to 60% of babies at some stage, usually at around 9 to 12 months. This is a period when you may be changing his nappies less frequently and also when his diet changes from milk only to a combination of milk and solids. Prolonged contact with urine and faeces can affect the baby's skin. Ammonia in the urine, and the acidity of the urine and faeces mixed together are the main culprits. Contact with these over a period of time can make healthy skin more susceptible to irritants, and this combination of a sensitive skin and exposure to irritants causes nappy rash.

Mrs North: What can be done to treat the rash and to stop it coming back?

Doctor: You can do a lot to prevent it and also to reduce the damage once it has started. As I explained, it is contact with a wet, soiled nappy that irritates the skin and brings on the spots. Check his nappy every hour and change it if it is wet or dirty. Wash the nappy area with water and keep it dry. You can apply barrier creams like Sudocrem or Drapolene to the nappy area. These are antiseptic emollients and I will supply you with some. Make sure that the skin is dry before you apply them. The most important thing to do is to expose his bottom to the air for as long as possible — try to do this three or four times a day. Avoid plastic pants which may irritate the skin. Avoid washing the nappy in strong detergents and biological powders and always rinse the nappy well, as any traces of washing powder are likely to make the rash worse.

If you do all this but the rash persists, contact your GP. Thrush sometimes causes a rash like this, and he may require treatment with an antifungal cream. A mild steroid cream may also be required to reduce the redness. Nappy rash can cause a lot of discomfort and Tim may get very irritable. You will have to be patient and very careful about keeping the skin clean and dry.

Mrs North: If the rash disappears with the treatment what can I do to prevent it from happening again?

Doctor: Follow a simple 'clean and dry' strategy. Change his nappy frequently. When you change his nappy make sure you wash any stale urine or barrier cream away using warm water, a gentle baby soap, and cotton wool. Avoid baby wipes as much as possible as they may contain chemicals that can irritate the skin. Let him spend time without his nappy on — fresh air will do him a lot of good. Use barrier cream to protect his skin in the nappy area: Zinc and Castor Oil Ointment, BP, Vaseline, or Sudocrem are all readily available at the chemists. Avoid using talcum powder over the nappy area — it can form tiny clumps, particularly if mixed with urine and faeces, which can irritate the skin. Is there anything else you would like to ask me, Mrs North?

Mrs North: No, thank you, doctor.

Mr Meredith, a 68-year-old man, is being discharged from hospital after having a transurethral resection of the prostate (TURP). You are the SHO on the urology firm. Advise him on what he can and cannot do over the next few weeks.

Patients who have a TURP are usually in their late sixties and often have many forebodings, some real, some imaginary, but all unsettling. They will have many questions and will need considerable reassurance. Your patient will be anxious to have answers to questions like these:

- When will I be fully recovered from surgery?
- Are there any complications that can happen at home?
- Was the prostate cancerous?
- Can the urinary problems recur after surgery?

Doctor: Good morning, Mr Meredith. I see you are ready to go home.

Mr Meredith: Yes, doctor, I am delighted about that.

Doctor: Excellent. Perhaps we could have a brief chat about what may or may not happen over the next few weeks?

Mr Meredith: Yes, please. That is a very good idea.

Doctor: Last time we talked I explained to you that your prostate gland was enlarged and was causing an obstruction to the urinary flow, and that it needed to be resected. Well, you agreed and we have done that. I am delighted that you have recovered very well from the surgery and that you are now ready to go home.

However, there are a few things that you need to know. First of all, you may notice blood in your water during the next 2 weeks or so. This is common after this type of surgery. Now and again urine flushes out some of the blood left over from the surgery, so don't be alarmed by it. It will settle down. You may also notice that you have an urge to pass urine often. Again, this is also common and will settle down. After all, your waterworks will need some time to get back to their old routine. Make sure you drink a lot of fluids at home — that will keep your system flushed all the time. Within the next 3 or 4 weeks it should all settle down.

Mr Meredith: Is there a danger of getting urinary infections?

Doctor: Yes, you will be more prone to urinary infections. If you get pain, discomfort, or a burning sensation when passing urine, or if you have a fever, please see your GP. It is possible that you may require antibiotics for a few days.

Mr Meredith: What about sex?

Doctor: Avoid sex for the first 2 weeks or so until all the sex and water channels have fully healed up. Then you can get back to normal. The amount of ejaculate may be reduced. This is because sometimes after a TURP the ejaculate may backtrack into your bladder. But don't worry. This is not going to harm you in any way. Sometimes the ejaculate may be bloodstained but, again, this will settle down.

Mr Meredith: Will the prostate grow back and give me problems in the future?

Doctor: This is a possibility but it is unlikely to happen for a long time.

Mr Meredith: Was the prostate cancerous?

Doctor: That is very unlikely as the initial biopsies you had did not show any evidence of cancer. However, we really need to wait until the pathologist has had a proper look at the gland we removed. We will get a report from him and I will speak to you again.

Mr Meredith, try to take things easy for the next few weeks. Do not overexert yourself. Increase your physical activity gradually. Lastly, you should avoid driving as much as possible for the next 2 weeks. We will see you in the clinic in 6 weeks. Is there anything else you would like to ask me?

Mr Meredith: No, thank you.

Doctor: Take care then, Mr Meredith.

Brian Tapping, a 23-year-old man, has been admitted into a psychiatric hospital with psychotic symptoms. A diagnosis of schizophrenia has been made. His family is shocked. You are the SHO on the psychiatry ward and your task is to talk to his father, Mr Tapping, and explain the illness and its treatment.

Schizophrenia is a serious mental illness. It has profound psychological and social implications for the entire family. The examiner will be testing your knowledge of psychiatry, and assessing your communication skills and ability to show compassion, as well as your fluency in the language. You are not expected to give a long lecture on schizophrenia; rather you have to summarize the important points in answer to each question you are asked and convey complex information in a way that will be readily understood.

Doctor: Hello, Mr Tapping. Please come on in and take a seat. I need to talk to you about Brian.

Mr Tapping: Can you explain what this condition is? What I have heard about it is that it is a terrible mental illness.

Doctor: Schizophrenia is a common mental illness affecting about one person in every hundred. Many people think that schizophrenia means 'split personality' but this is not true — it is more a splitting of psychological functions. While some functions, such as the ability to communicate, are impaired, others, such as memory and mathematical abilities, are retained. It is therefore a condition where thoughts, feelings, and actions are disconnected. People with schizophrenia experience the outside world differently, their behaviour changes and appears bizarre to other people. Most patients do not even realize that they have an illness.

The symptoms of schizophrenia can be divided into positive and negative symptoms. Every person is different and every patient with schizophrenia has a unique set of symptoms. One of the positive symptoms is that patients feel that thoughts are being put into their mind or taken out by a powerful outside force. Their body may feel as though it has been taken over by an alien, supernatural force. Another is that patients may have hallucinations, the experience of hearing, smelling, feeling or seeing things that do not actually exist. Hearing 'voices' is particularly common. Some patients also have delusions which are strongly held but false beliefs. They may be paranoid, believing that others are plotting against them and so on. Negative symptoms are things like a lack of motivation — patients may be untidy and show no emotional responses such as excitement or pleasure. They lack interest in life and often show a tendency to move downwards in social class.

Mr Tapping: What causes it?

Doctor: Schizophrenia is a very complex disease. The cause of this illness is not entirely understood but several factors are believed to play a role. Genetic factors may be significant and there may be several genes involved. Changes in the chemical composition of the brain may be responsible for the symptoms. It is also thought that parts of the brain may not have developed fully in some patients with schizophrenia. This may be due to complications during birth or to a viral infection during the early stages of pregnancy. Stressful life events can also trigger the onset of schizophrenia. It is also possible that some drugs of abuse, for example marijuana, ecstasy, or LSD, can trigger schizophrenia or make it worse in some people.

Mr Tapping: Will he recover from this or will he be in hospital for the rest of his life?

Doctor: I am afraid the prognosis in schizophrenia is rather poor. Although we have drugs we can use to control symptoms there is no specific treatment for this condition. In the short term, the more prominent the patient's positive symptoms, the more likely he is to recover from the acute episode. In the long term, say over a 30-year period, one-third of cases show some recovery or remission. Another third of patients recover from their initial episode but then go on to have relapses with some good periods of near normality in between. Unfortunately, one-third of patients will suffer a chronic form of the condition and may have to spend most of their lives in hospital.

There is a very good chance that Brian, who has predominantly positive symptoms, will recover completely from this episode and he is unlikely to be in the hospital for a long time.

Mr Tapping: What is the treatment?

Doctor: The initial treatment, as you will realize, will be in hospital. He will be observed and carefully assessed. As he is unaware that he has an illness and as he is a danger to himself and to others at the moment, he has been compulsorily admitted to the hospital under a section of the Mental Health Act. This can remain in force for up to 6 months at which time the situation would have to be reviewed.

We have started him on medication to control his symptoms — with several of the newer drugs that are available, it is usually possible to control these. There is a risk that his symptoms might come back if he stops his medication, however, and he will need to be on long-term drug therapy. This is just one part of treatment — he will also need a lot of support from his family and friends.

Once he recovers from the initial illness other services, like supported housing, day care, and employment schemes, will play an important role in his rehabilitation. He will also need significant input from the community mental health teams. For some patients with prolonged illness, specialist rehabilitation services, including residential care, may be required. There is no single treatment for schizophrenia. It requires a multidisciplinary approach.

Mr Tapping: Are Brian's sisters and brother at risk of developing schizophrenia?

Doctor: Yes, I'm afraid that it has been found that siblings are at higher risk of developing schizophrenia than the general population. However, at the present time it is not possible to quantify that risk exactly.

Mr Tapping: Are there any support organizations that we can join?

Doctor: There are a lot of support organizations for patients with mental illness, and their families and carers. It can be very upsetting when someone close to you has a schizophrenic illness. Patients can find the symptoms very frightening and after they recover from the initial episode they may feel guilty, ashamed, distressed, or angry. The National Schizophrenia Fellowship, or NSF, manages community self-help groups in various part of the country that offer support and advice for families. The Voices Forum, which is a part of the NSF, manages local self-help groups for sufferers of the illness. Associated with these groups is a network of community-based projects, including day-care centres, supported accommodation schemes, drop-in projects, and employment initiatives. SANELINE is a helpline for patients and families that offers advice and support. You may have already heard of MIND, a charity organization which provides useful information for patients and their carers.

There is a lot of support, help, and advice available. Here is a leaflet that gives you the addresses and contact phone numbers of all the relevant organizations. Is there anything else you would like to ask me?

Mr Tapping: No, thank you, not at the moment.

Doctor: In any case, while Brian is here you will be visiting him. So, if anything occurs to you please ask the charge nurse and he will find me. For the time being, goodbye.

Mr Mackay is a 60-year-old chronic smoker. He is being discharged from hospital after a serious bout of bronchitis. You are the SHO on the medical ward and your task is to advise him to stop smoking.

You should bear in mind that the intention to stop smoking is not a novel concept to most smokers and this patient, like most smokers, will not need (and may not like) a lecture on the subject. A more pragmatic approach might be to explore and expand what he knows already about the ill-effects of smoking, and to talk about the advantages of not smoking. Before advising the patient about a strategy for giving up, you should find out if he has already considered the idea himself, or if he has already tried and failed. You should explore the method he tried and why he failed.

Doctor: Good morning, Mr Mackay.

Mr Mackay: Hello, doctor. So, when am I going home?

Doctor: Well, how about today?

Mr Mackay: That would be great.

Doctor: As you know you came into hospital with a bad attack of bronchitis. You needed strong antibiotics, oxygen, nebulizers and chest physiotherapy. I am delighted that you have made a good recovery and that you are now fit to go home. Now you will have to make sure that your chest doesn't get any worse, or you will certainly go on to have more of these attacks. Have you any idea about what you could do to stop this happening?

Mr Mackay: I think I know what you're getting at. My own doctor has been at me a few times and I have tried to give up the cigarettes.

Doctor: So you do know that smoking is bad for you. Do you know how and why that is?

Mr Mackay: Well, for one thing I wouldn't be in this state if I had never smoked.

Doctor: Quite right! But that is only the beginning of the list. Smoking increases the risk of lung cancer, throat cancer, bladder cancer, kidney cancer, heart disease, peptic ulcer disease, chronic bronchitis, and other chronic lung diseases. Smoking not only puts *you* at risk, but also your family. It has been shown recently that your family at home will also inhale the smoke — this is what is called 'passive smoking'. If you have a baby at home, passive smoking could impair her mental and physical development and young babies are also at risk of the sudden infant death syndrome. Even the adults are at risk of developing heart and lung disease from passive smoking. Think about these risks to your family. People who die of diseases caused by smoking lose, on average, 10 to 15 years of their life. Stopping smoking reduces all these risks.

In your situation, if you do not quit smoking, there is a good chance that the bronchitis will get worse and give you more problems. I'm sure that you would not want to end up as a respiratory cripple, unable to breathe, and unable to walk around easily.

Mr Mackay: Hmm … Will stopping smoking reduce these risks immediately?

Doctor: Not immediately, but think about all the extra money you can save by not smoking. You will feel a lot healthier and will be able to breathe more easily when you exercise. You will smell fresher and you won't have bad breath and stained teeth and fingers. Your taste buds will become keener so your food will taste better. You will have less frequent fevers, colds, and chest infections. Your children and grandchildren will be less likely to start smoking and you will reduce any risk of health problems for the rest of your family. These days, sixty is not considered to be old and you will have less chance of having all those other conditions I mentioned if you remain a non-smoker for more than 5 years.

Mr Mackay: I see your point, doctor, but how can I stop smoking? I tried before with no success. All my friends smoke so it is very difficult to go out with them and not smoke.

Doctor: The most important thing is to decide to give up smoking once and for all, and to stick with your decision. Believe that you can do it. Stopping smoking all at once is better than gradually cutting down. Get rid of all the ashtrays, lighters, and cigarettes the night before you stop smoking. It is a good idea to find someone else who is stopping and do it together. If you feel the urge tell yourself that you can have a cigarette after the next meal but when that time comes put it off to the next meal, and so on. You need to keep your hands and mind off cigarettes. Perhaps this would be a good time to try a new hobby to distract yourself.

In this hospital, we have a counselling scheme for smokers, run by a trained nurse and supervised by a consultant. I have spoken to her about you and she would be happy to enrol you and provide regular counselling and support. She tells me that they have a 30% success rate among smokers referred from within the hospital. This compares very well with the general population, of whom only 2% of smokers manage to stop smoking each year. If you have the motivation they will build on that.

Mr Mackay: What about the withdrawal effects? I have been smoking for so many years!

Doctor: In addition to craving for a cigarette, you may feel irritable and find it difficult to concentrate. Some people feel sick and shaky. You may not get all of these symptoms but if you do get problems our anti-smoking counsellor will give you nicotine patches, inhalers, or lozenges. There is a new drug called bupropion which is a non-nicotine preparation. When this drug is given as part of a special scheme, like the one I am recommending to you, it can be quite effective in helping patients to stop smoking.

Keep working at it. Stopping smoking is not a passive process. Keep telling yourself why you are doing this. Save the money you could have spent so that you can see it growing. Work together with your family and friends and of course we are also here to help you.

Mr Mackay: Doctor, I think you have made up my mind. Thank you.

Doctor: You will be hearing from our counsellor, Mrs Davies, very soon. Take care, Mr Mackay. Do contact us if you have any new problems. As planned, we will see you in the clinic in 6 weeks and I will be keen to know how you are getting on.

Mr Paterson is a 75-year-old gentleman who lives alone in his flat. He is admitted for an inguinal hernia repair. You are the surgical SHO and your task is to explain the procedure and possible risks to Mr Paterson, and obtain consent from him.

A surgical operation, no matter how minor it seems to the surgeon, always causes the patient a lot of anxiety. Patients are often worried about the possible risks of surgery and its potential complications. They may also wonder if the condition might settle in time without surgery, or at least if the operation could be deferred. You should explain what a hernia is and how it is repaired as well as the potential complications of both the condition and the surgery.

Doctor: Hello, Mr Paterson. I am Dr Malik, Mr Freeman's Senior House Officer. He is the consultant surgeon. As you know you have been admitted today for a repair of the hernia in your groin.

Mr Paterson: Oh, hello, doctor. That's right. Mr Freeman said he would fix my hernia.

Doctor: Our House Officer, Dr Norman, has seen you and she asked you lots of questions about your general health, the medicines you take, and any surgery you may have had before. She also examined your heart and lungs and the hernia.

Mr Paterson: Yes, I saw another doctor earlier who gave me a full examination.

Doctor: Mr Paterson, I am going to explain a bit about the hernia, how we are going to repair it, and about any complications that could arise. Do you have any idea what a hernia is?

Mr Paterson: I know it is a lump that keeps coming and going and gives me a dragging ache in my groin.

Doctor: Yes, it is a lump caused by a protrusion of part of the bowel through a weak spot in the abdominal wall, which is either due to a congenital defect or to a weakness coming on later in life. This usually shows up as a lump, which at first is reducible — in other words, it can be gently pushed back into the tummy — but it can become troublesome if it is not repaired.

Mr Paterson: That's right, doctor. It does go back when I lie down, but it does ache sometimes, especially if I stand for a long time or walk any distance.

Doctor: Yes, at the moment you have a reducible hernia but it could become fixed and irreducible. The bowel could then become trapped and strangled. If that happened the bowel could become rotten and infected. Surgical repair at that late stage causes many complications. That's why we have advised you to have surgery now.

You will be having an anaesthetic and the anaesthetist will see you a little later on and explain more about that. The surgery entails a cut on the side of the hernia, about 10 cm long. Then we repair the hernia and reinforce the weak muscles with synthetic gauze. This will significantly reduce the chance of it coming back again.

Mr Paterson: Might there be any complications?

Doctor: Complications that can happen soon after the operation include pain, bleeding, urinary retention, haematoma or a blood clot, infection, and, occasionally, a clot in the leg. The late complications include recurrence of the hernia, and numbness or pain at the operation site. Very rarely there can be damage to the blood supply to the testicle, the blood vessels in the groin, or the bowel that is in the hernia. However, these are very rare complications.

We will make sure that we give you enough painkillers to control the pain. Gentlemen of your age can have temporary problems with passing water after any operation in the groin. Should that happen, we could put a catheter in for a while. You will have special stockings to wear and injections of a blood-thinning drug in the skin of your tummy to minimize the chance of any blood clots forming in your legs. You may need to have antibiotics if we suspect there is any infection, but the chances of this are very small. Very rarely a blood clot at the site of the operation may need to be cleared out. Any numbness or pain around the wound usually improves with time and the use of the synthetic gauze does significantly reduce the chances of a recurrence of the hernia.

Mr Paterson: How long does the operation take?

Doctor: It usually takes about 30 to 40 minutes. After surgery you will be in the recovery area until you are awake and more settled. Then you will be taken back to the ward. Depending on which type of anaesthetic you have, you will be able to start drinking and eating quite soon. It will be a bit sore initially but you will be given painkillers. In a day or two you will be up and around but we will only discharge you once you are comfortable, particularly as you live on your own.

We will make arrangements for the district nurse to keep an eye on the wound. The stitches are dissolvable and the dressing can come off in 2 to 3 days. You could then have a shower. It is quite common to have some swelling and discoloration of the wound and this may last for a week or two, so don't worry unduly about that. Once it has settled down you may feel a ridge under the scar. This is also normal and may take a few months to go completely.

Mr Paterson: When will I be able to drive?

Doctor: You can drive after a week, as long as you are able to make an emergency stop without feeling any pain. You can return to normal activities whenever you feel comfortable to do so but avoid heavy lifting and very strenuous activities for 5 to 6 weeks. Now, Mr Paterson, do you understand what a hernia is, what can happen to it if it is left untreated, and what we are going to do? We can't do any surgery on you without your written permission and you shouldn't sign anything unless you understand everything fully.

Mr Paterson: Yes doctor, you have explained everything, thank you.

Doctor: That's fine. Now, I would like you to sign this consent form. That gives us your permission to do the operation. The things I explained are also on this leaflet, which you can read later. Do come and ask me any questions that may occur to you later. Now, I am going to put a special identification mark on the side and position of the proposed operation.

Mr Gordon is a 30-year-old man who has come to the surgical outpatients department requesting a vasectomy. His wife has accompanied him. You are the surgical SHO and your task is to discuss it with them.

This couple probably know something about vasectomy as they seem to have come to a joint decision about having the operation. However, they may have some misconceptions or anxieties that you will need to address.

Doctor: Hello! Good morning, Mr and Mrs Gordon. I am Dr Kalra, Senior House Officer to Mr Webster, the consultant surgeon. I have read the letter sent in by your GP, Dr Lewis. I understand that you feel that you have completed your family and that you would like to have a vasectomy.

Mr Gordon: Yes, doctor. We have completed our family and are thinking of moving on to a more permanent method of contraception, such as a vasectomy.

Doctor: Right. I'll discuss that procedure with you but, before I do that, perhaps I can go over some of the details about you and your family with you. Your doctor tells me that you have two sons, of 7 and 5, and a 2-year-old daughter. Are they all healthy?

Mrs Gordon: That's right, doctor. They are all very healthy. They have had no problems apart from the usual childhood illnesses.

Doctor: So, you are quite happy with your three children. I also gather that you yourself are fit and well, Mr Gordon, and that you do not take any regular medication and have never had any surgery in the past.

Mrs Gordon: Yes doctor. He has had no health problems in the past. In fact, this is the first time he has been to a hospital so he is rather anxious!

Doctor: I am sure anybody coming to hospital for the first time would be anxious, especially for surgery. You both may have heard about vasectomy, but I am sure that you will be keen to know a bit more about it.

Mr Gordon: Yes doctor, would you please go through it with us.

Doctor: The operation involves making two small cuts on either side of the scrotum and then cutting out a small segment each of the two tubes that carry the semen from the testes to the penis. These tubes are called the 'vas deferens'.

Mr Gordon: Is it a reversible operation doctor?

Doctor: Vasectomy is irreversible as we cut out a small segment from each tube and tie off the ends. Of course, a reconstructive reversal of this operation is possible but the success rate is rather low, probably less than 50%.

Mr Gordon: Will I have an anaesthetic, doctor?

Doctor: Yes, in most patients we perform this operation under local anaesthesia and they tolerate it very well. This involves injecting a local anaesthetic into the skin of the upper part of the scrotum where we are going to make the incisions to take out the small segments of the tubes. The first prick is the worst part because it stings but once the local anaesthetic starts working you will not feel any pain. Of course, during the operation you will be aware of a little pulling and pushing. One of our nursing staff will be talking to you to divert your attention and the surgeon will also be asking you from time to time if you are feeling any discomfort or pain. However, if you'd rather, this can also be performed under a general anaesthetic.

Mr Gordon: Which do you think is better, doctor?

Doctor: As I said, the majority of patients prefer the local anaesthetic for its convenience — you don't have to fast beforehand and you can eat soon after the operation. However, general anaesthesia is also safe and you won't know anything about the operation, so you can choose whichever you wish.

I should point out to you at this stage that every surgical operation does carry some risks and complications, however small the risks may be. Early complications that can follow this operation are bleeding, formation of a blood clot, and infection. Possible late complications are failure of the vasectomy, lumpiness at the site of the operation, and sometimes a degree of pain, but all these are very rare and, of course, very difficult to predict.

Mrs Gordon: Doctor, would the operation affect his manliness, if you know what I mean?

Doctor: Only that he wouldn't be able to father a child which, after all, is the purpose of the operation. No, it will not affect your performance as a man in any sense, Mr Gordon. In particular, it will not affect your virility. Does that answer your question?

Both: Yes doctor. Thank you.

Mr Gordon: How long does the operation take, and do I have to stay in overnight?

Doctor: Usually the operation takes about 10 to 20 minutes and is done as a day case. You come to the day ward at the scheduled time and you would be discharged after the operation, once you're comfortable and have had something to eat and drink. You need to take it easy for just a couple of days. You may need to take simple painkillers for a few days. Once you are able to move about freely at home you can go back to work. Most men go back to work about a week after the operation.

Mr Gordon: Does the operation work immediately?

Doctor: No. You will have to use another form of contraception until two semen samples are negative for sperm. These will be done by your GP after 16 and 18 weeks. The consultant, Mr Webster, will write to you once he gets all the results of your tests.

Mrs Gordon: How will you know that the operation has been successful?

Doctor: Vasectomy is a very successful operation and the failure rate is less than 1%. We routinely send the segments of the tubes to the pathology laboratory to confirm that the correct structure has been divided. Also, the sperm tests will tell us if the procedure has worked.

Mr Gordon: What will happen if the tests show that the operation has not worked?

Doctor: As I have mentioned, the chances of failure are very small but if the tests confirm that the operation has failed, I am afraid we would have to repeat it. If that happened we would get you in quite quickly.

Mrs Gordon: We'll keep our fingers crossed! Thank you Dr Kalra. You've explained everything very well.

Doctor: Thank you, Mr and Mrs Gordon. This may all be too much to take in at once and you may think of some more questions when you get home. One of our team will see you in the day-case ward when you come in and they will be more than happy to answer any other questions that you might have.

Albert Penny, an 82-year-old gentleman, was admitted to your ward with pneumonia. Two days later he suddenly collapsed and died. You are the SHO on the ward. You would like a hospital postmortem examination to find out more about the cause of death. You need to talk to his bereaved wife, Mrs Penny, to seek her permission for this.

Hospital postmortems are also called 'interest postmortems' and are carried out by the pathologist without involving the coroner. Such postmortems are important not only because they inform us about the cause of death, which may have been unrelated to a patient's current illness, but also because they expand our knowledge about the evolutionary process of various diseases. In our enthusiasm for obtaining this information it can be all too easy to forget that the next of kin (who must give permission for a postmortem) is trying to cope with the loss of their dear one while we are explaining the need for the postmortem.

When you are talking to Mrs Penny you must remember her grief and be ready to console her. When you are trying to get consent for a postmortem it may be better not to ask for it at the outset, allowing the subject to come up during a conversation about the illness.

Doctor: Good morning, Mrs Penny. I am Dr Anand, the Senior House Officer on the ward. We met when Mr Penny was admitted. I am very sorry about the death of your husband but I'd like to assure you that he did not suffer. He passed away suddenly and peacefully.

Mrs Penny: It was such a shock to me. He seemed to be getting better when it happened. *(She will probably be tearful.)*

Doctor: Believe me, it was a shock to us as well, particularly as we thought that we were getting on top of his pneumonia. He seemed to be just about turning the corner.

Mrs Penny: Yes doctor. He looked all right when I left but no sooner had I reached home than they rang. By the time I got here he was dead. (*You will need to pause here to console her.*)

Doctor: I am very sorry. We tried very hard to revive him but we failed. He suddenly collapsed and in spite of all our efforts his heart would not start again.

Mrs Penny: What do you think happened? Why did his heart stop so suddenly?

Doctor: It is hard to tell. It could be that he had a heart attack or a clot in the lung. (*Pause.*) We would like to know what happened at the end. I am sure you would, too. (*Pause.*) The only sure way of finding out would be by doing a postmortem.

Mrs Penny: Oh no, doctor. I wouldn't want him to be opened up or mutilated.

Doctor: I understand your fear. It is quite understandable but I can assure you that it is not much different from a surgical operation. The pathologist opens up, looks at various organs and stitches the wound up very carefully. No evidence of the postmortem would be visible when he is in the coffin so he wouldn't look different in any way.

Mrs Penny: That's another thing. About the organs. I have read about doctors keeping body parts after a postmortem. I wouldn't want that to happen to my Bert.

Doctor: Yes, I'm afraid the medical community has received some bad press lately. But I can assure you that we wouldn't keep any organs unless it was absolutely necessary to look at them further to reach a proper diagnosis. If we need to study any organ in detail and have to keep a part or the whole organ, then either the pathologist or I would come back to talk to you. Of that I can assure you.

Mrs Penny: Bert always said that he wanted his body to be used to help others. It does upset me somewhat but you have eased my mind a lot and I would like to respect his wishes and let the postmortem go ahead. How long will it take?

Doctor: Thank you, Mrs Penny. It doesn't take long to carry out a postmortem, only an hour or so. It will probably be done tomorrow so that it won't delay the funeral arrangements.

Mrs Penny: I appreciate that you took the time to explain things to me, and thank you for looking after him.

Doctor: Once again, I am sorry that we could not save him. Our only consolation is that we tried very hard. If there is nothing else you would like to ask, could you just sign here please?

Mrs Penny: Yes, OK.

Mr Stokes, a 60-year-old man, has been referred with a cataract in his right eye. You are the SHO in the ophthalmology clinic and you need to talk to him about the cataract and the treatment options.

Cataracts are the commonest cause of blindness worldwide and of great concern to many elderly patients as they pose a threat to their independence. Mr Stokes may have many misconceptions about cataracts and cataract surgery and he is likely to ask you:

- What are cataracts?
- Do I need an operation?
- What are the risks?

Doctor: Good morning, Mr Stokes. I am Dr Tibbs, SHO in ophthalmology.

Mr Stokes: Hello, doctor. Thank you for seeing me. My optician tells me that I have a skin over my right eye. What does she mean?

Doctor: What your optician means is that the lens in your right eye is becoming cloudy and it does not transmit light as well as it did when it was shiny and crystal clear. This is called a 'cataract' and it prevents light getting through to the back of your eye. Objects in front of your eye cannot be seen clearly now at the back of your eye or in your brain.

Mr Stokes: How did I get it?

Doctor: Cataracts are a natural consequence of ageing — just as the skin or any other part of the body changes with age, so does the lens. It gradually becomes harder and loses its transparency. About half of all people aged over 65 have some degree of cataract.

Mr Stokes: Does this mean that I have to have an operation? The optician mentioned something about it not being 'ripe' yet.

Doctor: A ripe cataract is one in which the entire lens is opaque but these days we do not have to wait until a cataract is at this stage. Cataracts can be removed at any stage. If you are happy with your vision at the moment and are able to do all the things that you enjoy doing such as reading, watching television, or keeping up with any hobbies that you may have, then there is no need to have an operation.

Mr Stokes: If I don't have the operation will it get worse?

Doctor: Cataracts tend to progress at different rates in different people. Some can become very cloudy over just a few months while others change very little over many years.

Mr Stokes: My wife is disabled and I need to be able to drive. Am I legally allowed to drive with my eyesight as it is now?

Doctor: The vision in your left eye is still very good so you are still legal for driving.

Mr Stokes: You mentioned hobbies earlier. I enjoy model making and reading and I have found them more difficult lately. Would glasses help me?

Doctor: Occasionally glasses may improve things slightly but your optician has not been able to improve your sight much, despite changing your prescription.

Mr Stokes: What does the operation involve, doctor?

Doctor: This operation is usually carried out as a day-case procedure under a local anaesthetic. This means that you will be awake during the operation, which usually takes between 20 and 25 minutes. The cataract is broken up into small pieces by an ultrasound machine and removed through a small incision of 3 to 4 mm. After the cataract has been removed an artificial lens is implanted in the eye to help you focus after the operation.

Mr Stokes: Are there any risks?

Doctor: In the vast majority of cases, approximately 95%, there are no complications. However, it is an operation and complications can always arise. Thankfully, most of these are relatively minor and will not affect the outcome of the surgery. In a small number of cases a complication may arise that could make the vision worse than it was before or, very rarely, may result in loss of the eye.

Mr Stokes: Can a cataract come back?

Doctor: No, a cataract cannot recur because the entire lens is removed. During the operation a thin membrane is left behind the implant and in about 50% of cases this membrane can become cloudy and cause the same visual problems as a cataract. The treatment for this is a procedure called YAG capsulotomy, where a laser beam is used to make a small hole in the membrane to allow the light to get through.

Mr Stokes: Will I need glasses after the operation?

Doctor: We normally try to focus the eye for distance vision and so you may need glasses to help you read because the implant can't change its shape or strength as the natural lens can when it is focusing.

Mr Stokes: Do I have to decide just now?

Doctor: No, of course not. Cataract operations are not without their risks, even in the best hands, and should not be undertaken lightly. Think about it and if you think of any more questions do not hesitate to ask me. Here is a leaflet that may answer some or all of your questions about cataract surgery. It gives our direct-line phone number and you can get me through that. If you decide to have the operation let us know and we will put your name on the waiting list.

Mr Stokes: Many thanks for your help, doctor. Goodbye.

Doctor: Goodbye, Mr Stokes

Mrs Forrest, a 36-year-old lady, has been diagnosed with stage IB cervical cancer. Talk to her about treatment options.

Treatment for cervical cancer may involve surgery, radiotherapy, and chemotherapy, either alone or in combination. It largely depends on the stage and grade of the tumour:

Stage I (cancer confined to the cervix)

Stage IA (microscopic invasion, <5 mm penetration)

- Cone biopsy (proceed to radical hysterectomy if lymphovascular invasion on histology)
- Simple hysterectomy

Stage IB (macroscopic invasion, >5 mm penetration)

- Radical hysterectomy ± radiotherapy (if pelvic lymph node positive)
- Radical radiotherapy

Stage II (beyond cervix but within pelvis)

Stage IIA (upper vagina)

- Radical hysterectomy ± radiotherapy ± chemotherapy

Stage IIB (parametrium)

- Radical radiotherapy ± chemotherapy

Stage III (spread to lower third of vagina or pelvic wall)

Stage IIIA (lower third of vagina)

- Radical radiotherapy ± chemotherapy

Stage IIIB (pelvic wall)

- Radical radiotherapy ± chemotherapy

Stage IV (spread to other organs)

Stage IVA (bladder or rectal involvement)

- Radical radiotherapy ± chemotherapy

Stage IVB (distant spread)

- Chemotherapy
- Other palliative measures

Obviously the preferred treatment for this patient would be radical surgery or radical radiotherapy. You will have to discuss both of these forms of treatment in detail. She may ask the following questions during the consultation:

- What kind of cancer is it?
- What does the stage of cancer mean?
- What kind of treatment will I be offered?
- Are there any side effects?
- What is the outlook for me?

Doctor: Good afternoon, Mrs Forrest. I am Dr Khan, Senior House Officer in gynaecology.

Mrs Forrest: Good afternoon, doctor. Thank you for seeing me.

Doctor: You will remember when you first came with bleeding from the front passage that I asked for your permission to do a colposcopy and a biopsy, and mentioned the possibility that it might be a growth.

Mrs Forrest: Yes doctor, I remember. Is it cancer?

Doctor: Yes, I'm afraid the biopsy showed a cancerous growth of the neck of the womb, the cervix. It is a squamous cell carcinoma, the commonest type of cervical cancer. But a good sign is that the cancer is of low grade. You also had a CT scan which showed that it has not spread beyond the cervix. Based on these tests we think the cancer is stage IB.

Mrs Forrest: What does that mean?

Doctor: It means that the cancer, though it has penetrated through more than 5 mm of cervical tissue, is confined to the cervix. The good news is that this is curable.

Mrs Forrest: That is a great relief. What sort of treatment will I need?

Doctor: Well, there are two options — removal of the womb by surgery, or radiotherapy. Previous clinical trials have shown no difference in survival between patients treated either with surgery or with radiotherapy. This means that we need to have a detailed discussion about each type of treatment and their potential side effects and benefits. You will need to choose the form of treatment that suits you best.

Mrs Forrest: I see. Please go on.

Doctor: Let me talk about surgery first. The operation is called a radical hysterectomy. This essentially involves the removal of the womb, or uterus, the cervix, part of the vagina, the fallopian tubes, peritoneum, lymph glands, and possibly one or both ovaries. You would be in hospital for 5 to 6 days. The operation is usually performed under general anaesthesia, which means you will be put to sleep during the surgery and would not feel a thing. Sometimes we can perform the operation under spinal anaesthesia, which involves an injection into the spine. An anaesthetist will, of course, speak to you in much more detail nearer the time. Generally speaking, most patients sail through either type of anaesthetic with no major problems.

Right after the surgery you will have a tube, or catheter, passed through the urethra into the bladder. This will allow drainage of your urine as you may have difficulty passing water for the first day or two after surgery. You will also be given fluids through a drip into one of your veins during the first 24 to 48 hours. I will discuss all this with you again if and when you choose this option.

Mrs Forrest: What are the long-term side effects of having a hysterectomy?

Doctor: A hysterectomy can affect you physically, emotionally, and sexually. The most important thing to remember is that most patients sail through the surgery. It can take up to 6 to 8 weeks to recover completely from the operation and some ladies can take up to 12 months. You may feel weak and tired for several weeks. You will not have any more monthly periods and will not be able to have a baby of your own. If both ovaries are removed your body will become deficient in the female hormone, oestrogen, and this causes menopausal symptoms such as hot flushes and sweating, although these can be controlled to a great extent by hormone replacement therapy. Some patients feel depressed for a few weeks which is perfectly normal. There are a number of support organizations that can help you through this difficult period. You can resume normal sexual activity about 6 weeks after the operation. Some patients find that they have a reduced sexual drive after hysterectomy but some find it has quite the opposite effect. Here is an information sheet about hysterectomy. You may also like to contact CancerBACUP or the Hysterectomy Association for further information and advice.

Mrs Forrest: What about follow-up?

Doctor: You will be seen in the clinic 2 weeks after discharge. This is to assess your recovery from surgery and to discuss the pathology report. If there is any indication that the cancer may have spread beyond the cervix you may be referred for radiotherapy. This is to make sure that the cancer does not come back again.

Mrs Forrest: What about radical radiotherapy?

Doctor: Well, as I said before, the survival rate is the same for radical radiotherapy as for hysterectomy. Radiotherapy is essentially a high-energy X-ray treatment. There are two types of radiotherapy treatment used for cervical cancer: external or internal. In external radiotherapy the radiation comes from outside the body and is focused onto the area affected by the cancer. It is an outpatient form of treatment. The affected area will first be marked using X-rays and CT scans. This means that you will have to attend a planning clinic in the Radiotherapy Department. The radiotherapy field will be marked on the skin too. You will be given appointments to attend Outpatients for 4 to 5 weeks to have radiotherapy. Each session of treatment lasts for a few minutes. Once the external treatment is completed you will have internal radiotherapy and for this a small pellet of radioactive material will be inserted near the cancer for a short time. You have to stay in hospital for a little while for this.

Mrs Forrest: What are the side effects of the radiotherapy?

Doctor: You may notice some reddening and soreness of the skin during the later stages of treatment. Mild bleeding from the front passage, a burning sensation when passing water, diarrhoea, and tiredness are all common. These will settle down in a few weeks. Radiotherapy damages the ovaries permanently, causing menopausal symptoms, which can be controlled by hormone replacement therapy. A small proportion of patients may have long-term side effects from radiotherapy, affecting the bladder or the bowel. A burning sensation on passing water, blood in the stools and urine, and diarrhoea are some of these side effects. It is important to remember, however, that most patients do not have long-term problems with radiotherapy.

Here is an information sheet that explains radiotherapy. Have a careful read through these sheets and discuss it with your family. You have to choose the treatment that best suits you. Let me know what you have decided over the next 2 to 3 days so that I can arrange treatment. Is there anything else you would like to ask me?

Mrs Forrest: No, thank you, doctor.

Doctor: See you soon. Bye.

Mr Gray, a 62-year-old man, has been diagnosed as having a mesothelioma. Explain to his wife about the aetiology, the treatment options, and the prognosis.

Remember to obtain verbal consent from the patient before discussing clinical details with his relatives and friends. Understandably, Mrs Gray will be anxious and worried. Be empathetic and explain everything as clearly as you can. Avoid complicated terms and medical jargon during the conversation. Give her plenty of time to ask questions. She may ask some of the following questions:

- What is wrong with him?
- What is a mesothelioma?
- Is the cancer advanced?
- What treatment is available?
- What is the outlook?
- What other help is available?

Doctor: Good afternoon, Mrs Gray. I am Dr Roy, Senior House Officer in chest medicine.

Mrs Gray: Good afternoon, doctor. Can you tell me something about my husband's condition?

Doctor: Certainly. As you know, Mr Gray was admitted with shortness of breath on exertion and a right-sided chest pain. A chest X-ray suggested that there was fluid in the right side of his chest. To get a clearer picture we did a CT scan last week. This confirmed the presence of the fluid but it also showed some coarse thickening of the pleura, which is the layer that covers the lungs. The fluid is between the two layers of the pleura. To find the cause for this we took samples of the fluid and of the pleura for analysis. The biopsy was reported this morning and I'm afraid that it has shown a type cancerous growth which is known as a 'mesothelioma'. It is this mesothelioma that is responsible for Mr Gray's chest pain and shortness of breath.

Mrs Gray: What is a mesothelioma?

Doctor: As I mentioned, the lungs are covered by a specialized skin, or membrane, called the pleura. It has two layers, the outer and the inner pleura, and the space between them is called the pleural space. The pleura normally protects the lungs and produces a lubricating fluid which enables the lungs to move freely during breathing. It is lined by specialized cells called the mesothelial cells. For reasons that are not clearly understood the mesothelial cell can become abnormal and turn cancerous, leading to the growth of a mesothelioma. There are different types of mesothelioma, such as epithelioid, sarcomatous and mixed. Mr Gray has the epithelioid type of mesothelioma.

Mrs Gray: What causes a mesothelioma?

Doctor: The most important risk factor is exposure to asbestos. There are three types of asbestos — blue, brown, and white — and all three of them increase the risk of mesothelioma. Exposure to radiation and also to some chemicals, such as zeolite, a silicate mineral, also increases the risk. Recently, a possible link has been suggested between a virus, the SV40 virus, and mesothelioma. Polio vaccines given between 1955 and 1961 are thought to have been contaminated with this virus. Mr Gray used to work in the ship-building industry 30 years ago and I wonder if that might have exposed him to asbestos. It is important to realize, though, that people who have not been exposed to asbestos can also develop mesothelioma.

Mrs Gray: Is the cancer advanced?

Doctor: I'm afraid the CT scan showed that the cancer has spread beyond the pleura. It involves the lymph glands in the chest, the chest wall, and the lining of the heart, or pericardium. This is a fairly advanced, or stage III cancer.

Mrs Gray: Is it curable? Can you do anything about it?

Doctor: As the cancer has spread beyond the pleura it will not be possible to get rid of the tumour completely. However, a lot can be done to control the growth and to relieve the symptoms. We will be discussing Mr Gray's situation tomorrow when we have a meeting with the chest surgeon, the radiotherapist, and the medical oncologist. The treatment options include surgery, radiotherapy, which is a strong X-ray treatment, and chemotherapy, which means treatment with drugs.

In the first instance we will have to remove the fluid from the chest to relieve his symptoms. This is done by inserting a tube into the chest and draining off the fluid. Sometimes when we do this, the cancer cells leak through the drainage site and seed themselves onto the chest. To prevent this we may have to give some radiotherapy to the chest-drain site after the fluid has been drained and the tube has been removed. After tomorrow's meeting we may refer Mr Gray to our medical oncologist who will plan his further treatments.

Mrs Gray: Will the fluid build up again?

Doctor: I'm afraid so, although the timescale of this is almost impossible to predict. However, if the fluid does reaccumulate, we may have to drain it again and perform a pleurodesis. This means sticking the two layers of the pleura together by injecting a drug into the pleural space. Sometimes, we have to do this by means of an operation.

Mrs Gray: You mentioned surgery as an option to treat my husband's cancer. Could you explain that, doctor?

Doctor: Sure. There are two different types of operation, depending on the extent of the cancer. For patients whose tumour is limited to the pleura and who are medically fit, major curative surgery is feasible. On the other hand, in patients with more advanced disease, more limited surgery to remove the pleura and prevent fluid accumulation, and to relieve pain may be performed. Mr Gray may be suitable for this limited surgery if his symptoms continue despite other treatments. We will have to discuss this at our meeting tomorrow.

Mrs Gray: What about chemotherapy?

Doctor: Chemotherapy has a modest chance of shrinking the tumour. Several drugs have activity, either alone or in combination, including doxorubicin, cisplatin, and methotrexate. The timing of chemotherapy treatment depends on several factors and the medical oncologist will discuss this with you both in due course. New treatments are also being developed and tested all the time and Mr Gray may be eligible to participate in clinical trials testing new treatments for mesothelioma.

Mrs Gray: Will he need radiotherapy soon, doctor?

Doctor: Radiotherapy can help to control some of the symptoms such as the pain. We may have to keep this option for later on.

Mrs Gray: Do you know how long my husband has got?

Doctor: Mesothelioma is a difficult disease to treat. Different patients respond differently to treatment. It is impossible to predict the outcome in individual patients. An expert oncologist will be looking after Mr Gray and he will have the best treatment available. He will be seen regularly over the next few months and every effort will be made to make him feel better.

Mrs Gray: Is there any other help available for my husband?

Doctor: Yes, there are lots of organizations that can provide valuable support. You could contact the British Lung Foundation and the British Thoracic Society for more information. There is a Mesothelioma Information Service at Cookridge Hospital in Leeds. CancerBACUP provides information, emotional support, and practical advice to patients and their carers. Here is an information sheet that gives you details of these organizations.

Mrs Gray: Thank you, doctor, for being so honest with me.

Doctor: Not at all, Mrs Gray. Please do not hesitate to contact me if you have any further questions. We will do all we can to make Mr Gray feel better and keep him comfortable. Bye for now.

Mr Russell, a 50-year-old man, has been suffering from stage IV non-Hodgkin's lymphoma for the past 5 years. He is known to have a para-aortic mass and is now complaining of back pain for which he has been taking co-dydramol, but with little benefit. You are the SHO in oncology. Explain further management, particularly with regards to pain control.

Pain in cancer may have several causes:

- Compression of surrounding tissues by progressive cancer
- Spread of cancer to other areas, e.g. bones
- Tissue damage caused by treatment (surgery, radiotherapy, chemotherapy)
- Infection
- Emotional factors — stress, anxiety, depression

This 50-year-old man is likely to have had several types of treatment, including chemotherapy and, possibly, radiotherapy. Pain control in this patient will require a multidisciplinary approach. If the pain is due to progressive disease, then it may be controlled by further chemotherapy or radiotherapy. Referral to a pain clinic or palliative care team may be justified where an effective analgesic regime can be drawn up. Finally, the patient may benefit from referral to the psycho-oncology service for the management of any emotional issues.

This patient is likely to ask you what is causing his pain. He will want to know what other treatments or painkillers are available, and what their side effects are. Lastly, he might ask if any other help is available.

Doctor: Good morning, Mr. Russell. I am Dr Raj, the Senior House Officer in oncology.

Mr Russell: Good morning, doctor. I am having an awful pain in my back. What do you think is causing it?

Doctor: As you know, you have had four different chemotherapy treatments for your lymphoma over the past 5 years. The cancerous lymph glands are in several areas, including the neck, armpit, chest, and in your tummy, next to the big blood vessel, the aorta. These glands around the aorta, the para-aortic lymph nodes, have increased in size and because they overlie the spine they are pressing on it and giving you pain in your lower back.

Mr Russell: Can anything be done for it?

Doctor: I'm sure it can. I see you have been taking co-dydramol tablets regularly for the past 4 weeks and though you had some benefit at first, the pain has now become worse. We will have to reconsider how to control it. A combination of radiotherapy over these glands and a stronger painkiller would be the best option. First, let's talk about the painkillers. We need to use a stronger painkiller and the drugs we use most commonly are morphine and morphine-like drugs.

Mr Russell: I thought morphine has a lot of side effects, doesn't it?

Doctor: I'm afraid powerful remedies have powerful effects, both desirable and undesirable, but most patients on morphine medication experience no major problems. We usually start with a low dose and then build up gradually to get the best control. This ensures that you get the pain control you need with the minimum of side effects.

Mr Russell: What are the side effects?

Doctor: Morphine can cause drowsiness, which usually settles in a few days as you get used to the drug. It can make you feel tired as well. Constipation is a common side effect, but this can be controlled with other medications — you may have to take a regular dose of laxatives. Some patients may feel sick. This can also be controlled with tablets. A dry mouth is another common side effect but as long as you drink plenty of fluids it should not be a problem.

Mr Russell: What if I get *all* the side effects?

Doctor: Unlikely, but if it does happen we can try other morphine-like drugs that cause fewer side effects. These include fentanyl, methadone, oxycodone, and hydromorphone.

Mr Russell: How is morphine given?

Doctor: Morphine is available as short-acting and long-acting tablets, syrup, soluble granules, and suppositories. It is a good idea to start with a short-acting formulation. The tablet form is called Sevredol and is available as 10 mg tablets. The liquid form is called Oramorph. Initially you can take the medication as and when you require it. Once we have an idea of how much morphine you need a day, we can work out the dose you need of the long-acting medication, which is taken twice a day, morning and evening.

Mr Russell: Is morphine available as an injection as well?

Doctor: Yes, diamorphine, a relative of morphine, is available in an injectable form. It can be given as an injection under the skin, into a vein or into a muscle.

Mr Russell: Is there anything that I should not do while taking morphine?

Doctor: Avoid alcohol, as it is likely to increase the drowsiness. Avoid working with heavy machinery, and it is advisable not to drive if you feel drowsy. You should contact the DVLA for further advice. You must also keep the tablets in a safe place, out of reach of children.

Mr Russell: Is there any other medication that I can take?

Doctor: Yes, in fact I would like to start you on a tablet called diclofenac. You have to take this twice a day. It can be particularly good for bone pains. It is usually well tolerated but can sometimes causes indigestion and, occasionally, stomach ulcers. You can minimize these side effects by taking this tablet after meals. We may have to give you other medications if indigestion is a problem.

Mr Russell: What about other sorts of treatment?

Doctor: Sure. As I said before, shrinking the tumour may relieve the pain. Radiotherapy is the next option. It is a high-energy X-ray treatment that would be given only to the glands that are pressing on the spine. It has fewer side effects than the drugs and there is a good chance that it could control your pain. We will be referring you to the radiotherapist who will discuss this with you in detail.

Mr Russell: Thank you.

Doctor: Is there anything else you would like to ask me?

Mr Russell: No, doctor.

Doctor: I am sure that with all these treatments we have we can get on top of the pain and make you feel better. Do not hesitate to contact me if you have any other problems. Take care, Mr Russell. Bye.

Mrs Cowan is a 38-year-old lady and she is 16 weeks pregnant. She is very worried that she may be carrying a baby with Down's syndrome. You are the SHO in the antenatal clinic and she has come to see you with a view to having investigations.

Mongolism, now referred to as Down's syndrome, is the commonest single cause of mental handicap, occurring in 1 in 700 of all live births in most populations. The incidence varies with the age of the mother: at 25 years the incidence is 1 in 1400, increasing to about 1 in 46 at the age of 45 years. This lady, at 38 years, is understandably worried about her 1 in 175 risk of having a baby with Down's syndrome. She will want to know if this risk can be investigated with clear-cut results and if the investigations themselves have any side effects. You should allow her to express her concerns and then offer her reassurance and the appropriate investigations.

Doctor: Hello, Mrs Cowan. Good morning, nice to see you.

Mrs Cowan: Good morning, doctor.

Doctor: Now, I see you are 16 weeks pregnant and the midwife has already seen you and done all the necessary documentation and testing. She tells me that you have some special concerns about this pregnancy.

Mrs Cowan: Yes, doctor. You are right. You see this was unexpected. Don't get me wrong, it is not unwanted, just unplanned. Now all the fears of a pregnancy at my age are dawning on me.

Doctor: Mrs Cowan, you don't need to worry. We will monitor your progress throughout and ensure that your pregnancy and labour go as smoothly as they would at a younger age.

Mrs Cowan: I am not worried about pregnancy itself, just that at my age I might have a baby with Down's syndrome.

Doctor: Well, actually, the majority of babies with Down's syndrome are born to younger mothers, but it is true that you have a higher risk at 38.

Mrs Cowan: I thought so. Can you test me for this, doctor?

Doctor: Yes, certainly. There are a number of tests we use, involving both invasive and noninvasive techniques. Let me give you some general details before we discuss the particulars in your case. Screening for neural tube defects, such as spina bifida, and Down's syndrome is offered at 16 weeks. This is done by taking the mother's age into consideration and by measuring two hormones in your blood, α-fetoprotein and human chorionic gonadotrophin. Don't worry about these long names — we'll call them AFP and HCG for short. In pregnancies complicated by a neural tube defect the AFP is elevated, and in pregnancies complicated by Down's syndrome the AFP is reduced but the HCG is elevated.

Ultrasound scanning can also be used in the first trimester to measure the amount of thickening over the back of the neck of the fetus. Increased translucency in this area has been associated with a greater risk of chromosome abnormalities. This can diagnose up to 80% of Down's syndrome babies. Using all these noninvasive approaches together, detection rates of approximately 90% can be achieved, but there is a 5% false-positive rate as well. In other words, in one hundred such tests the diagnosis of Down's syndrome may turn out to be wrong in five cases.

So much for the noninvasive tests. There are two invasive tests, amniocentesis and chorionic villus sampling, or CVS, that can be performed at 14 weeks' gestation. The CVS test can be performed even earlier in pregnancy and has a detection rate of approximately 70%, again with a 5% false-positive rate. I'm afraid apart from this possibility of making the wrong diagnosis, there is also a risk of miscarriage, of about 1%, associated with the invasive tests.

I am sorry, this is rather a lot to take in but I will give you a printed sheet that gives you all this information. You can take it with you and study it, and also discuss it with your husband.

Mrs Cowan: Thank you, doctor. You have been a great help in explaining all this to me. I'll take this with me to remind myself of the tests you have gone through with me.

Doctor: I will do the blood tests for AFP and HCG today and I will arrange the ultrasound as well. The results should be available within a few days and, in the meantime, you can think about having the amniocentesis or CVS. Both these tests are particularly useful for DNA analysis and the diagnosis not only of Down's syndrome but also other inborn errors of metabolism.

Mrs Cowan: Yes, doctor, I would like to have the blood tests done today. If I want to have CVS done, when can that be arranged?

Doctor: I will have to bring you in for a day or two for that but I can arrange it within the next few days, perhaps towards the end of the week. Let's meet again in 3 days' time when I will have the results of today's tests.

Mrs Cowan: That will be fine. Thank you, doctor.

Mr Havers, a 62-year-old man with severe osteoarthrosis of his knee joints has been admitted for a right knee replacement. You are the SHO in orthopaedics and you have to obtain his consent for this operation.

The prospect of any operation will be a mixture of anxiety about the procedure and hope that it will improve things, particularly when the patient has significant symptoms such as pain or difficulty in walking. Mr Havers will have some idea about the operation from his discussions with the consultant, but he will need to have the details of the operation and aftercare explained to him in fairly simple language.

Doctor: Hello, Mr Havers. I am Dr Malik, Mr Leinster's SHO — he is the consultant who is going to operate on your knee. Dr Evans, our ward doctor, has already examined you and written up all your details. I am here to have a brief chat with you about the operation and to get you to sign this consent form. You probably have some idea what the procedure entails?

Mr Havers: Yes, Mr Leinster said that he was going to fix me up with a new knee joint.

Doctor: Not entirely. He will fix some new parts onto your old knee so that you will have no pain and you will be able to walk about more freely than you have done for the past few months.

Mr Havers: Will it last as long as the old one did?

Doctor: Well, you know, man can't match nature but I daresay it should be good enough for anything between 12 and 16 years.

Mr Havers: What exactly will he do?

Doctor: The procedure is called the 'universal condylar replacement' and it is aptly named because it is universally tried and trusted! The operation will last for just under 2 hours but you will be put to sleep and you won't know a thing. The anaesthetist will come to see you today to have a word with you. Once you are out, Mr Leinster will make a cut, about 10 to 12 cm long, on the front of your right knee and expose the bones of the joint. As you have had osteoarthrosis for a long time, the opposing surfaces of the bones, where they hinge with each other, are rough and worn out. He will clean out the joint, remove the rough edges, and fix on three components — the femoral component is fixed onto the bottom edge of the thigh bone, the patellar component onto the kneecap, and the tibial component onto the top edge of the lower leg bone. He will make sure that the joint surfaces are well aligned and functional before he closes the wound.

Before the operation you will have some antibiotics and a mild sedative. After the operation you will rest in bed for the first 48 hours. We will give you a blood-thinning agent so that you don't form any clots in your legs. Our physiotherapist will get you moving again, starting with the quadriceps exercises on the day after the operation, when the drains come out. This means simply straightening the leg several times a day. The walking will start after 3 to 5 days, first with a zimmer frame, then with two crutches, and finally with a stick. She will also teach you some exercises to bend and straighten your knee. If bending the knee proves difficult they will put you on a machine which bends your knee for you until it becomes free and mobile. You should be able to go home by the weekend but, remember, you will have to keep doing the exercises because the knee muscles go thin very quickly if you don't use them. You will come back here the following week when we will remove the stitches, and we will see you again 2 weeks after that for another X-ray and a check-up. Remember, rehabilitation is a continuing programme and we will keep a regular check on you. Do you understand now what is involved?

Mr Havers: Yes, doctor. More or less.

Doctor: Well, if you have any questions you can ask me now, or if anything occurs to you later you can always ask to see me again.

Mr Havers: I think I've got the gist of it.

Doctor: In that case, perhaps you would be kind enough to sign this form. By signing it you are giving us your permission to operate on you. Please read it carefully. It states that I have explained the procedure and that you have understood it.

Mr Havers: I'm quite happy to sign it, doctor.

Doctor: Thank you. Now I must put an indicator mark on your right foot to identify the correct side for the operation. We wouldn't want them to operate on the wrong knee, would we?

Mr Havers: No, doctor, certainly not!

Doctor: All the best. See you later.

Mr Hutchins, a 60-year-old man, had a barium enema as an outpatient and has been admitted now for a colonoscopy. You are the SHO in the gastroenterology firm and you are seeing him in order to obtain his consent for the procedure.

It is clear that Mr Hutchins is under investigation for a complaint affecting his lower bowel and should therefore have some idea about what a colonoscopy is and why it has been arranged. He may also have made some enquiries amongst his friends and acquaintances about the procedure and possibly its complications. It is always important that the doctor seeking the consent of a patient for a procedure should know its indications, contraindications and possible complications.

Indications

Diagnostic
- Abnormal barium enema suggesting a colonic polyp or other neoplasm
- Lower bowel haemorrhage
- Diverticular disease with chronic symptoms
- Follow-up of patients with previous polyps or cancer
- Lower bowel symptoms with a negative barium enema
- Inflammatory bowel disease (to assess the extent and for biopsy)

Therapeutic
- Removal of polyps
- Cauterization of vascular dysplasia

Contraindications

- Acute ulcerative colitis
- Acute diverticulitis

- Ischaemic bowel disease
- Radiation colitis
- Peritonitis
- Pregnancy

Complications

- Rupture of the bowel
- Haemorrhage
- Retroperitoneal emphysema

Doctor: Good morning, Mr Hutchins. I am Dr Lal, the SHO to Dr Platt, who will perform the colonoscopy. I presume you know something about the procedure.

Mr Hutchins: Yes, I can remember some of what Dr Platt explained to me. I was under the impression that it would be an outpatient job.

Doctor: Well, the procedure itself is fairly straightforward in expert hands but the preparation is very important and that is best undertaken in hospital. You see we need to empty your lower bowel so that we can get a good look at it. You will be kept on a liquid diet for the next 2 days and we will give you enemas on both days to empty the bowel. Besides, we may have to consider doing more investigations, which can be done more easily while you are in hospital. If there are no other tests to do you can go home after a few hours' rest after the colonoscopy.

Mr Hutchins: That is something to look forward to after 2 days of starvation and enemas! Would you remind me briefly about the procedure?

Doctor: It is something like the sigmoidoscopy you had before but, instead of a rigid tube, this time they will be using a flexible tube that goes further up the bowel. It is fitted with a camera so that what the operator sees can be photographed and projected onto the screen. This way there is a good chance that the source of your bleeding can be identified. The passing of the tube into your back passage will cause some discomfort but they will use enough lubrication to make it as painless as possible. They will also give you an injection of diazepam before the procedure to relax you — that will help you as well as Dr Platt when she tries to negotiate the tube up into the bowel.

Mr Hutchins: Are there any complications to be wary of?

Doctor: Colonoscopy is not free from risks, though in most cases there are no problems. Even though it is a flexible tube, undue pressure can, very rarely, cause rupture of the bowel. There is sometimes a minor haemorrhage or a leakage of gas from the bowel into the surrounding tissues. However, Dr Platt is an old hand at this procedure and I do not anticipate any problems. Is there anything else you would like to ask?

Mr Hutchins: No, Dr Lal. Thank you.

Doctor: I have to obtain your written consent for this procedure. Please read this form and then sign it at the bottom. It states that I have explained the procedure, that you have understood my explanation, and that you have no objection to us proceeding with the colonoscopy.

Mr Hutchins: That's fine. I will sign it.

Doctor: Thank you. Bye for now.

Clinical examination

Introduction

This will not be a new exercise for you as most of you will have had to take clinical examinations at different stages through medical school and all of you will have had to pass them in the final year. The purpose here, as it was in your final exams, is to test your ability to carry out a physical examination of a system (e.g. chest, heart, abdomen) or a subsystem (e.g. visual fields, thyroid, knee, breasts). There are a few differences between this exam and your final exam, however. Many of you may not have any experience of the objective structured clinical examination (OSCE) format. As we explained in earlier sections, at any particular station there is the same task, the same time to do it in, the same patient, and the same examiner with the same preprinted mark sheet, for each candidate. These constraints make it a much fairer test than the traditional format but it does also introduce some degree of artificiality for the candidates and tedium for the examiners. The other difference is that you will mostly see a 'patient' who is usually an actor who has been trained to display the same signs to each candidate (e.g. peripheral neuropathy, a visual field defect). Also, some of the examinations, such as that of the breasts, may have to be carried out on a manikin and you must show the same delicacy and respect as you would display to a real person.

We have presented 27 examination routines in this section and these cover almost everything that you may be asked to do. You should practise them on manikins and on colleagues so that you become spontaneous and dextrous, performing all the steps in the correct sequence. It is dangerous to think that as you have done them all before you can reproduce them when the time comes. You should practise them all several times over so that the stress of the exam does not wipe them from your memory.

Exam etiquette

- Carefully study the rules and regulations given in the GMC's *The PLAB Test, Part 2, Advice to Candidates*, and follow them. For example, do not forget to bring the appropriate proof of identity, and do not enter or leave a station unless the bell rings.
- Introduce yourself to the patients and be gentle and courteous at all times. Do not forget that each patient will be examined

along the same lines, repeatedly, by a number of candidates. Try not to hurt them, cover each part after the examination, and do not forget to thank them at the end.

- You may be tested on your record-keeping, so do not forget or underestimate the importance of details that may seem trivial to you, such as your name, date, time, and the patient's name. Make a careful note of your findings.
- Do not forget to thank the examiner when you are finished. They have to maintain their alertness to do a fair job and it can be very tiring.

Please examine this patient's heart.

The subject to be examined may be a manikin, a healthy volunteer, or a real patient with a diagnosable lesion in the cardiovascular system. The examiner may give you a short history and then ask you to examine the heart, the cardiovascular system, or a part of it. It is worth remembering some of the conditions that might be present if the subject happens to be a real patient:

- Mitral stenosis
- Mitral regurgitation
- Mixed mitral valve disease
- Aortic stenosis
- Aortic regurgitation
- Mixed aortic valve disease
- Combined mitral and aortic valve disease
- Congenital heart diseases, e.g. VSD, PDA, ASD
- Coarctation of the aorta
- Prosthetic heart valves

Examination

Approach the patient from the right side and have a brief introductory chat with him, 'I am Dr Shamir. I have been asked to examine your heart. May I?' In the exam the patient will probably be wearing a gown but if he is wearing a shirt, ask him to remove it so that the chest and neck are exposed for your inspection.

Inspection

Start with a quick but comprehensive visual survey of the patient. Observe whether he is comfortable or in distress, and if there are any of the following signs:

- Pallor
- Cyanosis
- Breathlessness
- Jaundice
- Facial pigmentation (e.g. bronze discoloration in haemochromatosis; slate-grey appearance with amiodarone therapy; telangiectasia in carcinoid syndrome)
- Malar flush (mitral stenosis)
- Clubbing of the fingers or toes
- Skeletal deformities (e.g. ankylosing spondylitis and rheumatoid arthritis, associated with aortic regurgitation)
- Pedal oedema
- Tall and lanky stature (Marfan's syndrome, associated with aortic regurgitation)
- Bruising (? warfarin therapy)

Look at the neck for pulsations, which may be forceful carotid pulsations (coarctation of the aorta, Corrigan's sign in aortic incompetence), or tall, sinuous venous pulsations (congestive cardiac failure, tricuspid incompetence, pulmonary hypertension). Look at the chest for any scars of old surgery and for any pulsations which might indicate left ventricular overactivity.

Palpation

Pulses

Count the pulse for at least 15 seconds to get a reasonable idea of its *rate, rhythm, volume,* and *character.* If it is a large-volume pulse find out if it is *collapsing* by lifting the arm and feeling for an abrupt flick over the radial, and the brachial or axillary arteries (Fig. 4.1.1). If the pulse volume is small (mitral stenosis, aortic stenosis) you should determine if it is *slow-rising* (aortic stenosis) by feeling the brachial and the carotid (Fig. 4.1.2). Ask yourself whether the rhythm is regular or irregular: if irregular, whether it is regularly irregular as in frequent ectopics; or irregularly irregular as in atrial fibrillation.

Feel the opposite radial pulse and look for the femoral pulse (Fig. 4.1.3) to check for *radiofemoral delay* (coarctation of the aorta). Next, look and feel the pulsations in the neck to confirm the impressions gained from inspection. Corrigan's sign (vigorous rise and quick fall of the carotid pulsation) will complement the presence of a collapsing pulse, which you may have already discovered. Look for any prominent visible

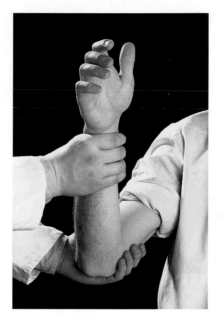

Fig. 4.1.1 Testing for a collapsing pulse

pulsations. Determine if they are venous or arterial. Jugular venous pulsations are better seen than felt and they have a wavy character; fall on inspiration; increase with pressure applied to the abdomen (*hepato-jugular reflux*); can be obliterated by

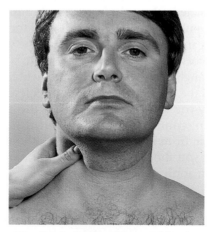

Fig. 4.1.2 Feeling the carotid pulse

251

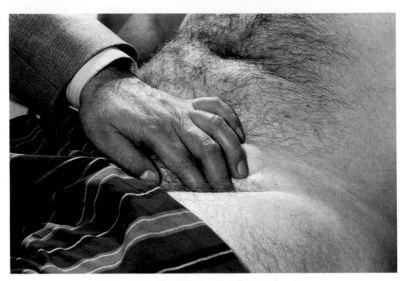

Fig. 4.1.3 Feeling for the femoral pulse

pressing on the root of the neck; and their height changes with the position of the patient.

This is also the time to identify the individual waves of the venous pulse by timing them against the opposite carotid pulse, coordinating what you see with what you feel. A large *v wave*, which coincides with the carotid pulse and sometimes even 'pulsates' the ear lobe, suggests tricuspid incompetence. In such a patient you should, later on, demonstrate a pulsatile liver by gently placing your knuckle in the right hypochondrium. Prominent *a waves* are seen in pulmonary hypertension and tricuspid stenosis and *cannon waves* are seen as sharp knocks in the venous pulse in complete heart block. Measure the height of the venous column from the sternal angle using two rulers, one held upright at the sternal angle and the other across at the upper level of the venous column. This way you will be able to express the height of the venous column in centimetres (the normal height with the patient at 45° is 3 to 4 cm from the sternal angle). Although unlikely in the exam setting, you should look for any pulsations of the trachea (*tracheal tug*, as in aortic arch aneurysms).

Precordium
Place the palm over the precordium to localize the apical impulse (Fig. 4.1.4). Once you feel the apical impulse, usually in

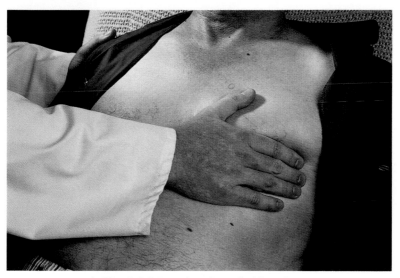

Fig. 4.1.4 Locating the apical impulse

the lower and the outermost region of the precordium, stand your index finger on it to determine the point of maximum intensity (PMI) and to appreciate the character of the impulse. Note the position of the apex with respect to the mid-clavicular line and the intercostal spaces, counting from the second space which lies against the sternal angle. The impulse can be graded as *just palpable*, *lifting* (diastolic overload as in aortic or mitral incompetence), *thrusting* (stronger than lifting), or *heaving with sustained lift* (outflow obstruction as in aortic stenosis). While your hand is placed across the precordium you may feel a *tapping impulse* as a brief, evanescent tap (left atrial 'knock' in mitral stenosis) or *thrills* over the mitral area.

Place your palm over the right ventricular area and apply sustained and gentle pressure (Fig. 4.1.5). If there is right ventricular hypertrophy (pulmonary hypertension) or volume overload (congestive failure), you will feel and see the heel of your hand lifted with each systole. You may feel the knock of a *palpable P_2* (pulmonary hypertension) over the second left intercostal space. Palpate over the aortic area for any *thrills*. The systolic thrill of aortic stenosis is best felt if the patient leans forward with his breath held after expiration, with your palm over the aortic area. It is worth trying this manoeuvre if you have already noted a slow-rising pulse.

253

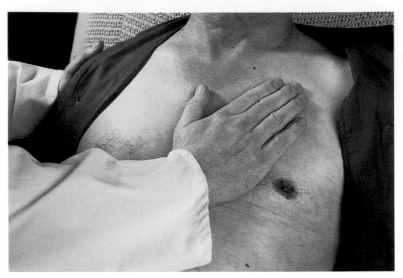

Fig. 4.1.5 Feeling for right ventricular heave

Percussion

This is of limited value in cardiovascular examination but it may be useful to percuss for any obliteration of the normal cardiac dullness over the left third and fourth spaces (absent in emphysema and dextrocardia). The right and left cardiac borders can be delineated with percussion, though this is more accurately done by radiography.

Auscultation

The success of auscultation lies in the art of selective listening, and that can only be done if you have meticulously gone through the preceding steps and so have a reasonable idea of what you expect to hear. There is always the possibility that there might be an auscultatory 'surprise', but the candidate who checks out the expected findings first has a better chance of detecting any surprises if they do arise.

Place the bell of the stethoscope lightly over the precordium and time the first heart sound, either with the apical impulse, if that is clearly visible or palpable, or with the carotid pulse. You should now be able to identify systolic and diastolic murmurs with confidence. You should listen for any expected murmurs in the most favourable positions. This is certainly necessary for the

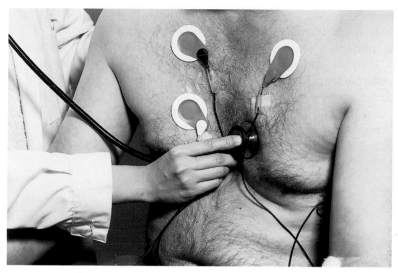

Fig. 4.1.6 Listening for an early diastolic murmur

early diastolic murmur of aortic incompetence (Fig. 4.1.6) and the mid-diastolic murmur of mitral stenosis (Fig. 4.1.7), two of the most easily missed murmurs. The early diastolic murmur is best heard with the patient leaning forwards, with the breath held after expiration, and the mid-diastolic murmur is more easily heard with the bell of the chest piece with the patient lying

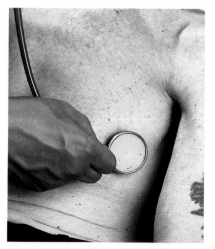

Fig. 4.1.7 Listening for a mid-diastolic murmur

255

on the left side. The early diastolic murmur is a high-pitched sound and, like all such sounds, is best heard with the diaphragm.

If the venous pressure is raised you should check for sacral oedema, listen over the lung bases for inspiratory crackles, and demonstrate a pulsatile liver, especially if you have seen a large *v* wave. If the instruction is that you should examine the cardiovascular system you should also feel all the accessible pulses and measure the blood pressure. If you have time you should offer to do this anyway.

Please examine the respiratory system of this patient.

The examiner might give you a few of the patient's symptoms (e.g. cough, breathlessness) before asking you to examine his respiratory system, but sometimes you are given a short and straightforward instruction like this one. The purpose here would seem to be that your examination skills for the whole system are being tested. In the examination of the respiratory system, all four components of examination (inspection, palpation, percussion, and auscultation) are used and your competence in using these skills can be tested in some depth. The subject may or may not have a respiratory disorder but you should consider the main possibilities:

- Pleural effusion or fibrosis
- Chronic obstructive airways disease
- Pneumonia
- Bronchiectasis
- Fibrosing alveolitis
- Old tuberculosis
- Pancoast's tumour
- Cor pulmonale
- Bronchogenic carcinoma
- Superior vena cava obstruction

Examination

You should not waste any time and appear as if you are thinking what to do. This patient or volunteer will already have consented for this examination and it is not necessary for you to obtain their consent, but a brief introductory remark (e.g. 'Hello, I am Dr Duroshola. I have been asked to examine your chest'.) is always a good start. The patient is often undressed and wearing a gown, but if not, you should ask politely that a shirt or blouse be removed. Do not help patients undress unless they specifically ask for your help. Set the backrest at 45° and ask the patient to recline and relax. During these initial pleasantries you should be starting your inspection routine.

Inspection

General
Look around and see if there is a sputum pot nearby (copious amounts suggest bronchiectasis) or a peak flow meter (chronic airways obstruction). Look at his general state for any evidence of *weight loss* (neoplasm, 'pink puffer'), distended veins on the chest and face (superior vena cava obstruction), and for *central cyanosis* (blue discoloration of *warm* parts). This is best detected by looking at the tongue and buccal mucosa in natural light. It may be due to cor pulmonale, fibrosing alveolitis or any condition in which there is central mixing of arterial and venous blood.

Upper respiratory tract
Observe if the patient is breathless, either at rest or from the effort of removing his clothes, and if he purses his lips or uses the accessory muscles when he breathes (chronic small airways obstruction, pleural effusion, pneumothorax). Look to see if the *cricoid–manubrium* distance (normally 4–8 cm) is reduced (chronic small airways obstruction); if the *neck veins* are distended; and if the *trachea* is central, which is sometimes quite easily seen (Fig. 4.2.1).

Breathing
Listen to the breathing (without the stethoscope) as you observe the chest for shape, contour, and movements, and the fingers for nicotine staining and *clubbing* (Fig. 4.2.2) (bronchial carcinoma, mesothelioma, pulmonary fibrosis, and suppurative lung disorders such as bronchiectasis, empyema, lung abscess). Listen carefully to see if expiration is prolonged (small airways obstruction), or noisy (breathlessness), and if there are any noises such as clicks (bronchiectasis) or wheezes (small airways obstruction).

Ribcage
The ribcage may be *hyperinflated* (Fig. 4.2.3) and moving mainly upwards (emphysema), or *asymmetrical* (Fig. 4.2.1) (fibrosis,

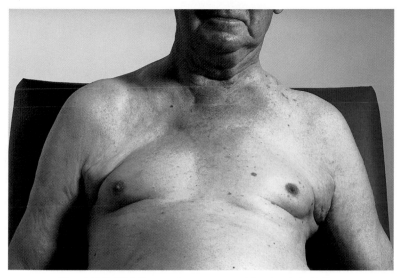

Fig. 4.2.1 Old thorocatomy scar and tracheal deviation

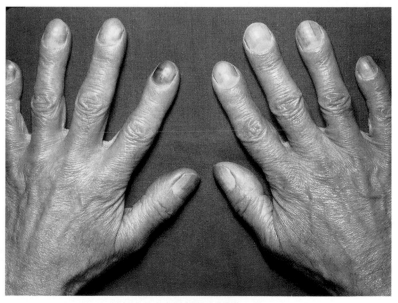

Fig. 4.2.2 Clubbing of the fingers

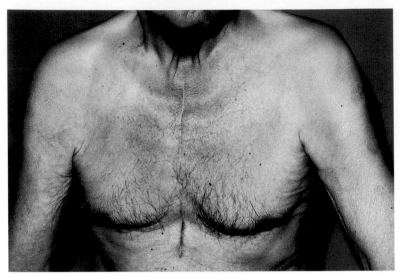

Fig. 4.2.3 Hyperinflated chest

pneumonectomy, collapse, pleural effusion, pneumothorax), and
there may be localized *apical flattening* (fibrosis due to old
tuberculosis), a thoracoplasty *scar,* or *indrawing* of the lower
intercostal spaces on inspiration (emphysema).

Palpation

Symmetry

Palpation, percussion, and auscultation are all carried out first on
the front and then on the back of the patient. Feel the pulse and
locate the apex beat (this can be difficult over a hyperinflated
chest) which, in conjunction with tracheal deviation, may suggest
mediastinal displacement (fibrosis, collapse, pneumonectomy,
effusion, pneumothorax). If you suspect *asymmetry* rest your hands
on either side of the front of the chest to see if there is less
movement on one side during inspiration.

Chest expansion

Next, grip the chest symmetrically with the fingertips in the rib
spaces on either side and approximate the thumbs to meet in the
midline in a straight line (Fig. 4.2.4). Observe whether or not the
thumbs move symmetrically from the midline and measure the
distance between them at full inspiration with a tape measure

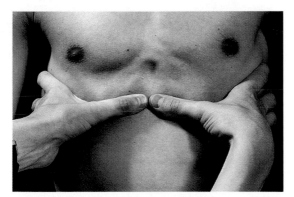

Fig. 4.2.4 Expansion shown by separation of the thumbs

(Fig. 4.2.5). The expansion should be measured both in the inframammary and the supramammary regions. It is better to use a tape measure to give you a more accurate assessment (Fig. 4.2.6). Palpate both axillae to detect any lymphadenopathy.

Trachea

Now feel the trachea with the middle finger while you place the index and the ring fingers over the prominent points of the manubrium on either side (Fig. 4.2.7). This procedure will give you a good idea whether the trachea is central or deviated to one side. If you have already found that the ribcage is hyperinflated and moving upwards, then feel for a *tracheal tug* (i.e. the middle finger being pushed upwards against the tracheal rings during inspiration by the upward movement of the chest wall)

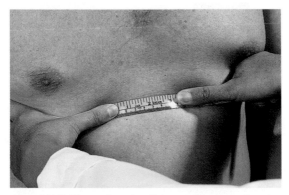

Fig. 4.2.5 Measuring the distance between thumbs

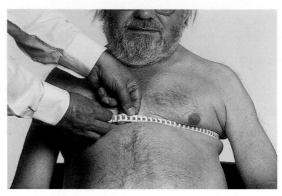

Fig. 4.2.6 Measuring expansion after full inspiration

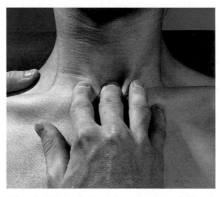

Fig. 4.2.7 Is the trachea in the midline?

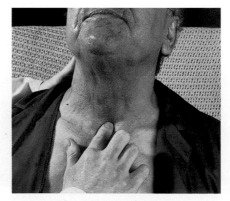

Fig. 4.2.8 Tracheal tug

(Fig. 4.2.8). *Be* gentle while you do this in case you cause the patient any discomfort (which would please neither him nor the examiner).

Vocal fremitus
Complete your palpation by checking for vocal fremitus by applying the ulnar aspect of the hand in each rib space (Fig. 4.2.9) from above downwards, asking the patient to say 'ninety-nine' at each contact.

Percussion

Percuss over the rib spaces from above downwards starting with the supraclavicular fossa and over the clavicles, but do not percuss over the bare bones in case this should cause discomfort to the patient. Do not forget to percuss over each axilla (Fig. 4.2.10). The normal cardiac and hepatic dullness may be lost over hyperinflated chests. The note obtained over a pleural effusion is *stony dull* like that elicited by percussing on a stone or brick wall (try this if you have difficulty in appreciating it). Apart from the excessive dullness of the note, the fingers will also feel some resistance from the chest wall.

Auscultation

Ask the patient to breathe gently through the mouth while you listen with the bell, starting over the supraclavicular fossae and moving downwards as you did for percussion, not forgetting the axillae. Apart from the fact that most respiratory noises are low-pitched, the use of the bell gives you an excuse in the exam to

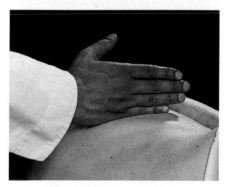

Fig. 4.2.9 Vocal fremitus

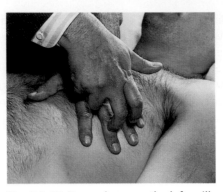

Fig. 4.2.10 Percussing over the left axilla

check your findings with the diaphragm! Also, harsh breath sounds heard with the diaphragm near a major bronchus (over the second intercostal space anteriorly or below the scapula near the midline posteriorly) may give an erroneous impression of bronchial breathing, particularly in thin subjects.

Complete auscultation by checking *vocal resonance* in all areas. Ask the patient to say 'ninety-nine' while you listen over each space, starting at the apices. The sounds resound in your ears if you listen over an area of bronchial breathing (*aegophony, bronchophony*). In such a case, you should also check for *whispering pectoriloquy* by listening over this area while the patient softly whispers 'sixty-six' — the sounds are heard clearly, as if spoken directly into your ears.

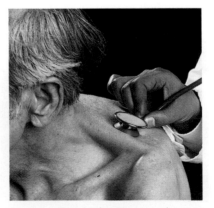

Fig. 4.2.11 Auscultation over the apex

To examine the back of the chest sit the patient forward and ask him to cross his arms in front of himself (to displace the scapulae laterally as far as possible). Now repeat your palpation, percussion, and auscultation, making sure that you do not forget to examine the apices (Fig. 4.2.11). You may also wish to palpate the neck to detect any lymphadenopathy.

Please examine this patient's abdomen.

The examiner may simply be wishing to see your technique, but you have to bear in mind that the subject may be a real patient and may have one or more of the following findings:

- Palpable liver or spleen or both
- Single palpable kidney
- Polycystic kidneys with/without a transplanted kidney in the iliac fossa
- Iliac fossa mass
- Signs of chronic liver disease
- Ascites
- Any other abdominal masses

Examination

Approach the right side of the patient and have a preliminary introductory chat. Ask her to lie supine on one pillow (if comfortable), with the whole abdomen and chest in full view and her hands by her side. Ask the patient to lower her clothes to a level about halfway between the iliac crest and the symphysis pubis.

Inspection

General
While these preparations are being made you should be performing a visual survey of the patient. The physical signs that you may observe in these few seconds include pallor, pigmentation, jaundice, spider naevi, parotid swelling, gynaecomastia, scratch marks, tattoos, abdominal distension, distended abdominal veins, an abdominal swelling, hernias, and decreased body hair. Even if the patient is an actor with no

abnormal signs you should be able to recall these signs. As the patient is getting into the correct position, quickly examine the hands for Dupuytren's contracture, clubbing, leuconychia and palmar erythema.

Pull down the lower eyelid to look for pallor. At the same time check the sclera for icterus and look for xanthelasma. The lower conjunctival fornix is the best place to look for pallor or for any discoloration (e.g. cyanosis, jaundice).

When they ask you to examine the abdomen many examiners would like (and expect) you to concentrate on the abdomen itself without delay, and yet they will not forgive you if you do not look for other, possibly associated, abnormal physical signs elsewhere. Never underestimate the importance of a good visual survey — a trained eye will miss nothing important on the face or on the hands while the patient is being properly positioned. That said, these initial observations need not occupy you for more than a few seconds.

Abdomen

Observe the abdomen in three segments (epigastric, umbilical, and suprapubic) for any visible signs such as pulsations, generalized distension (ascites) or a swelling in one particular area. Note any scars or fistulas (previous surgery, Crohn's disease). Look for distended abdominal veins (the flow is away from the umbilicus in portal hypertension but upwards from the groin in inferior vena cava obstruction). The examiners may want you to demonstrate how to determine the direction of the venous flow.

Palpation

Unless the examiner asks you to go straight to the abdomen, start palpation at the neck and supraclavicular fossae for cervical lymph nodes, which might suggest an intra-abdominal malignancy. If you do find lymph nodes you should examine the axillae and groins for evidence of generalized lymphadenopathy (lymphoma, chronic lymphatic leukaemia). As you move from the neck to the chest, you should check for gynaecomastia (palpate for *glandular* breast tissue in obese subjects), spider naevi (possibly already noted on the hands, arms and face, also may be present on the back), and scratch marks.

With practice the examination to this point can be completed very rapidly and will provide valuable information which may be overlooked if you rush straight on to palpation of the abdomen. If the examiner insists that you start with abdominal palpation it suggests that there is little to be found elsewhere but you should nevertheless be prepared to keep your mind and eyes open so as not to miss any relevant features.

Palpation of the abdomen itself should be performed in an orthodox manner — any temptation to go straight for a visible swelling should be resisted. Put your palm gently over the abdomen and ask the patient if he has any tenderness and to let you know if you hurt him. First, systematically examine the whole of the abdomen with *light* palpation. Palpation should be done with the pulps of the fingers rather than with the tips, the best movement being a gentle flexion at the metacarpophalangeal joints with the hand flat on the abdominal wall.

Next, examine specifically for the internal organs. For the liver start in the right iliac fossa and work upwards to the right hypochondrium (Fig. 4.3.1). Gross splenomegaly, reaching the umbilicus, would have been detected on the initial light palpation. If you have not found a huge and easily palpable mass arising from the left subcostal region you should start palpation for the spleen a few centimetres below the left subcostal rim (Fig. 4.3.2). The organs are felt against the radial border of the index finger and the pulps of the index and middle fingers as they descend on inspiration, when you can gently press and move your hand upwards to meet them.

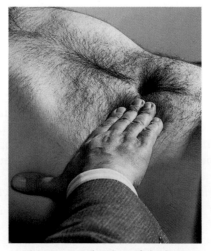

Fig. 4.3.1 Palpation of the liver

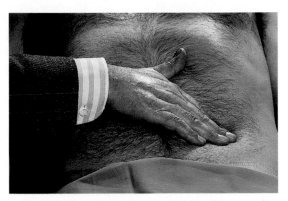

Fig. 4.3.2 Examining for moderate splenomegaly

The kidneys are then examined by *bimanual palpation* of each lateral region. Place one hand over the lumbar region, just below the costal margin and lateral to the rectus abdominis, and the other posteriorly, opposite it, with the fingers in the renal angle (Fig. 4.3.3). While the patient takes a deep breath press the flat of both hands towards each other — the lower pole of the descending kidney may be felt between the two hands.

If you see a patient in the examination with a mass in the left hypochondrium the examiner may ask you if you are sure that it is a spleen and not a kidney or vice versa. You will have to establish whether you can get above the mass and separate it from the costal edge, whether you can palpate it bimanually and if the percussion note over it is resonant (all features of an enlarged kidney).

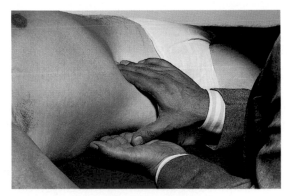

Fig. 4.3.3 Bimanual palpation

269

Palpation of the internal organs may be difficult if there is ascites. In this case the technique is to press sharply, flexing at the wrist joint, to displace the fluid and palpate the enlarged organ (*dipping* or *ballottement*).

Finally, palpate deeply with the pulps of your fingers to feel for the ascending and descending colons in the flanks; use gentle palpation to feel for an aortic aneurysm in the midline; and complete the palpation by feeling for inguinal lymph nodes, noting obvious hernias and the amount of pubic hair.

Percussion

This is done from the nipple downwards on both sides to locate the upper edge of the liver on the right and the spleen on the left. You should define the lower palpable edges of the spleen and liver by percussion in the orthodox manner — proceeding from resonant to dull areas.

If you suspect that there is free fluid in the peritoneum you must establish its presence by demonstrating *shifting dullness*. Initially, check for stony dullness in the flanks. There is no need to continue with the procedure for demonstrating shifting dullness if this is not present. By asking a patient with ascites to turn on his side you can shift the dullness and demonstrate this by percussing from the dependent, dull area to the top, where the note will become resonant.

Before you conclude the palpation and percussion of the abdomen, ask yourself whether you have found anything abnormal. If there appear to be no abnormal physical signs make sure that you have not missed a polycystic kidney or a barely palpable splenic edge, or, occasionally, a mass in the epigastrium or iliac fossa.

Auscultation

Auscultation usually has very little to add in the exam setting. However, as part of the full routine, you should listen to the bowel sounds, check for aortic and renal artery *bruits*, and listen for any other sounds, such as a rub over the spleen or kidney, or a venous hum (both extremely rare).

Examination of the external genitalia and a rectal examination are not usually required in the exam. However, you can conclude the examination by stating that you would normally complete your assessment by examining the external genitalia (especially in a male with chronic liver disease, who may have small testes; or if there are palpable cervical lymph nodes, as the drainage of the testes is to para-aortic and cervical lymph nodes) and the rectum.

Please examine this patient's arms.

This instruction is usually given only when there is something easily visible on the arms or when the examiner wishes you to perform a neurological examination of the upper limbs. It is useful to remember some of the conditions that can be diagnosed by inspection of a patient's arms:

- Psoriasis
- Lichen planus
- Herpes zoster
- Cellulitis
- Purpura
- Rheumatoid arthritis
- Neurofibromatosis
- Sclerodactyly

Bearing in mind that you may have to carry out a neurological examination, you should also be thinking of various relevant neuromuscular signs and conditions:

- Wasting of the small muscles of the hand
- Hemiplegia
- Muscular dystrophy
- Motor neurone disease
- Parkinson's disease
- Cerebellar syndrome
- Old polio
- Ulnar nerve palsy (claw hand)
- Carpal tunnel syndrome

Examination

Inspection

As always, inspection is the most important part of the examination. The information you gain not only may lead you to the correct diagnosis but might also direct your subsequent examination. It may be an obvious 'spot' case and you may not have to do anything more than just describe what you see. On the other hand, you may pick up a clue at this stage that would solve the mystery and relieve your anxiety about the diagnosis.

While you exchange greetings with the patient, look at the face for any asymmetry (hemiplegia), wasting (muscular dystrophy), a fixed, immobile expression (Parkinson's disease), or nystagmus (cerebellar syndrome). Look at the neck for loss of muscular bulk (muscular dystrophy); at the elbows for psoriasis, rheumatoid nodules, scars, or deformity (ulnar nerve injury); at the forearms for any skin lesions; and at the hands for any swelling, deformity, wasting, or tremor. If you see any wasting then you should look carefully for *fasciculation* which can be easily missed on a cursory inspection.

This process should take only a few seconds. If there is joint disease or a skin condition you should complete the examination by looking for all the relevant signs elsewhere in the body. For example, if you see any psoriatic plaques on the elbows you should look for pitting of the nails, erythematous lesions on the scalp, especially along the hairline, and psoriatic lesions on the trunk and knees. If you do not suspect a diagnosis requiring specific further examination, or have observed a neuromuscular sign, you should start a full neurological examination at this stage.

Neuromuscular examination

Although you would already have noticed any wasting, you should now systematically assess the *muscle bulk* in the upper arms, forearms and hands. Once again, look for any fasciculation. Test the *tone* by flexing and extending at the elbow and wrist in an irregular and unexpected sequence. Roll the wrist gently to see if there is *cog-wheel rigidity* (Parkinson's disease).

Ask the patient to stretch his arms in front of him and keep them up. Look for any winging of the scapulae. Ask the patient to close his eyes and watch for any sagging of the arm, suggestive of weakness, upward movement (cerebellar disease), or wandering of the fingers, suggestive of impaired joint position sense (cervical myelopathy).

Power

Next, test power, starting with abduction at the shoulder joint. This can be covered by asking the patient to carry out the following manoeuvres:

- *Deltoid, C5.* Raise your arms to the side (*demonstrate this to the patient with your arms at 90° to your body*) and stop me pushing them down.
- *Biceps, C5,6.* Bend your elbow: stop me straightening it (Fig. 4.4.1).
- *Triceps, C7.* Push your arm out straight and don't let me stop you (Fig. 4.4.2).

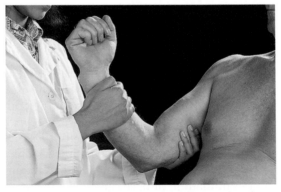

Fig. 4.4.1 Testing power in the biceps (C5,6)

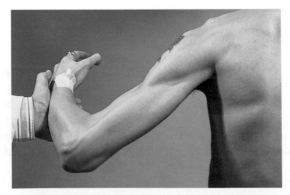

Fig. 4.4.2 Testing power in the triceps (C7)

- *C8, T1.* Squeeze my fingers (*hold out two fingers, one on top of another*) (see Fig. 4.10.10; p. 310).
- *C7, radial nerve.* Hold your fingers out straight (*demonstrate*). Now stop me bending them (Fig. 4.10.11; p. 310).
- *Dorsal interossei, ulnar nerve.* Spread your fingers apart (*demonstrate*). Stop me pushing them together (Fig. 4.10.12).
- *Palmar interossei, ulnar nerve.* Hold this piece of paper between your fingers and stop me pulling it out (see Fig. 4.10.13; p. 311).
- *Abductor pollicis brevis, median nerve.* Point your thumb at the ceiling (*demonstrate*), and stop me pushing it down (see Fig. 4.10.14; p. 312).
- *Opponens pollicis, median nerve.* Make a pinch with your thumb and little finger, and stop me pulling them apart.

Coordination
Test coordination by asking the patient:

- Would you like to tap on your chest? Do this as quickly as you can; now with the other hand; now with both hands
- Tap quickly on the back of your hand — right on left, then left on right, as fast as you can (*demonstrate rapid alternating movements*) (Fig. 4.4.3).
- Touch the tip of your nose with your index finger; now touch my fingertip (*ask the patient to run between the two while you vary the target. Note any clumsiness and past-pointing*) (Fig. 4.4.4).

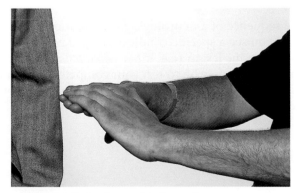

Fig. 4.4.3 Testing rapid alternating movements

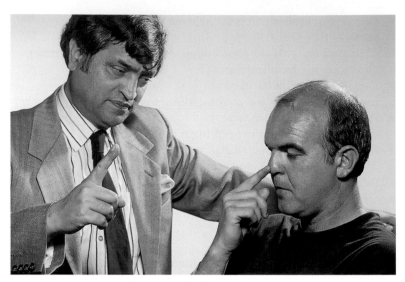

Fig. 4.4.4 The finger–nose test

Reflexes

Check the reflexes — biceps (C5,6), triceps (C7), and supinator (C5,6).

Sensation

Finally, test sensation, first *light touch* and *pinprick*, and then *vibration* and *joint position sense.* In all cases start over the fingers and then progress upwards, bearing in mind the dermatomes and the areas of sensation covered by the ulnar, median and radial nerves.

The entire sequence of a neurological examination may not be necessary if you see a specific condition (e.g. claw hand) or a sign suggesting a specific lesion (e.g. ulnar nerve palsy). However, the examiner's purpose may be to test your competence at carrying out a *full* examination, and he may not interrupt until you have completed your entire examination routine.

Please examine this patient's legs.

The examination of the legs, like that of the arms, could involve either an obvious spot case or a complete neurological examination. Among the possibilities that might be presented as a spot case, you should bear in mind the following signs and diagnoses:

- Oedema
- Ulceration (vasculitis, ischaemic, pyoderma gangrenosum)
- Knee or ankle swelling
- Vasculitis
- Purpura
- Erythema nodosum
- Diabetic foot
- Necrobiosis lipoidica diabeticorum
- Paget's disease
- Pretibial myxoedema
- Varicose veins
- Deep venous thrombosis
- Psoriasis
- Pemphigus, pemphigoid

Similarly, you should think of the various possible *neurological conditions*, and there may be a sign or a clue that may suggest that you should carry out either a limited or a full neurological assessment. Among the conditions that are commonly presented are:

- Peripheral neuropathy
- Hemiplegia
- Spastic paraparesis
- Motor neurone disease
- Cerebellar syndrome
- Charcot–Marie–Tooth disease

- Common peroneal nerve palsy
- Old polio

Inspection

Examination

Although the focus of the examination will be on the legs, you should not ignore the fundamentals of inspection and must start at the face, looking for any signs such as enlargement of the cranium (Paget's disease), asymmetry (hemiplegia), exophthalmos (pretibial myxoedema), or nystagmus (cerebellar syndrome).

Look at the arms for any evidence of rheumatoid disease or osteoarthrosis, wasting (motor neurone disease, Charcot–Marie–Tooth disease), and of fasciculation (motor neurone disease).

Look carefully at the legs, at the shape for any bowing (Paget's) or swelling (oedema, deep venous thrombosis); at the skin for any lesions (purpura, vasculitis, psoriasis) or signs of vascular insufficiency (shiny, pale skin, absence of hair, cyanosis, ulcers, or gangrene); and at the joints for any arthritis. If a lesion is visible a full examination may not be required: you will be able to describe the characteristic features and give the diagnosis. This is also the time to decide if there is vascular insufficiency, which will require a specific examination of the skin for temperature and capillary filling, and of the pulses.

You may have noted *pes cavus* (Charcot–Marie–Tooth disease, Friedreich's ataxia) or that one leg is smaller than the other (old polio, infantile hemiplegia), or found no obvious signs and suspect that a neurological examination is required. You should once again assess the overall muscle bulk. It is profitable to recall some of the neurological disorders with characteristic *muscle wasting* that are commonly seen in the exam, such as diabetic amyotrophy with anterior thigh wasting, Charcot–Marie–Tooth disease with distal muscle wasting, polymyositis with proximal muscle wasting, old polio with unilateral wasting, and common peroneal nerve palsy with lateral compartment wasting in the leg. During this survey, note if there are any *abnormal movements* such as fasciculation (motor neurone disease).

Neuromuscular examination

Tone

Examine tone by rolling the knee from side to side. In hypertonia the foot will waggle en bloc with the leg. Put your hand behind the knee and lift it rapidly and watch the heel. It will lift off the bed easily if hypertonia is present. Flex and extend the knee and plantarflex and dorsiflex the ankle rapidly to assess the resistance or tone.

Power

Next, test power by asking the patient to perform these manoeuvres:

- *Hip flexion (L1,2)*. Bring your knee up and stop me pushing it down.
- *Hip extension (L5,S1)*. Push your leg down towards the couch and stop me pushing it up (Fig. 4.5.1).
- *Hip abduction (L4,5)*. Push your legs apart against my hands (Fig. 4.5.2).
- *Hip adduction (L2,3)*. Bring your legs together and stop me pushing them apart.
- *Knee extension (L3,4)*. Bend your leg, and now straighten it against my hand.
- *Knee flexion (L5,S1)*. Bring your heel towards your bottom and stop me pushing it away.
- *Ankle dorsiflexion (L4,5)*. Cock your foot up and stop me pushing it down (Fig. 4.5.3).
- *Plantarflexion (S1)*. Press your foot hard against my hand.

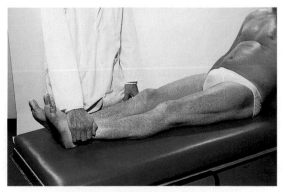

Fig. 4.5.1 Testing hip extension

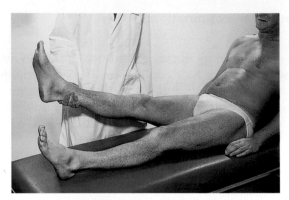

Fig. 4.5.2 Testing hip abduction

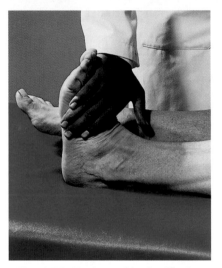

Fig. 4.5.3 Testing ankle dorsiflexion

Coordination
Test coordination by asking the patient to run his heel smoothly up and down along the opposite shin (see Figs 4.6.2 and 4.6.3; p. 285). You may also ask the patient to tap his foot quickly on your hand (see Fig. 4.6.4; p. 256).

Reflexes
Test the knee reflex (L3,4) (Fig. 4.5.4) and ankle reflex (S1,2). If there is hypertonia demonstrate ankle and patellar clonus. Test the *plantar response* by stroking the outer part of the heel with a

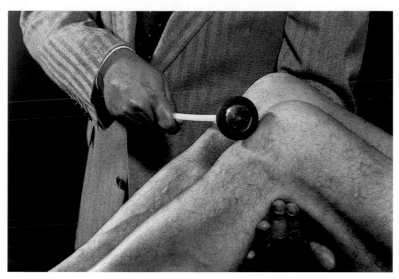

Fig. 4.5.4 The knee jerk

key or an orange stick, taking care that you do not hurt the patient.

Sensation
Test sensation, starting with *light touch* (dab cotton wool lightly), then *pinprick* (with a paper clip or a disposable pin), testing the dermatomes from the feet upwards. Complete the sensory examination by testing *vibration* and *joint position sense* (Fig. 4.5.5).

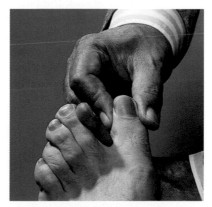

Fig. 4.5.5 Testing joint position sense

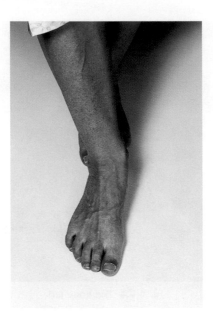

Fig. 4.5.6 Walking heel-to-toe

Gait

Examination of the legs is not complete unless you check the patient's gait. Check that the patient can walk and ask for his (and the examiner's) permission to examine his gait. First, watch his ordinary walk to a defined point and then ask him to walk 'heel-to-toe' (ataxia) (Fig. 4.5.6); on his toes; and on his heels.

Finally, perform *Romberg's test* by asking the patient to stand with his feet together and the arms outstretched. Stand near him and be ready to support him if there is any ataxia. Now ask him to close his eyes and see if he is more unsteady with the eyes closed. (Romberg is positive in sensory ataxia, e.g. tabes dorsalis, subacute combined degeneration of the spinal cord).

Please examine this patient's cerebellar system.

This involves examining the speech for *dysarthria*, the eyes for *nystagmus* and the arms, legs and gait for *incoordination*. The subject may be a normal volunteer but you should bear in mind that it may be a patient with one of the following conditions:

- Multiple sclerosis
- Cerebellar syndrome of malignancy
- Alcoholic cerebellar degeneration
- Brainstem vascular lesion
- Friedreich's ataxia
- Anticonvulsant drug toxicity

Examination

As you talk to the patient and ask for his permission to examine him, you may be able to detect *dysarthria*. Look at his eyes for any *nystagmus* or any limitation of movement of the eyeballs. In a patient with multiple sclerosis, there may be signs of weakness of one or more limbs. After the initial visual survey of the patient go on to examine the speech, eyes, limbs, and gait.

Speech

First, ask the patient some general questions, such as 'What is your name?', 'What is your address?' Then ask a few questions that require longer answers, such as, 'Tell me what you had for breakfast today' and 'Would you count from one to twenty, please?' Ask the patient to repeat after you, 'British Constitution' and 'West Register Street'. As the patient speaks, note if the speech is slurred, jerky, and explosive, suggestive of *ataxic dysarthria*. There may be inspiratory whoops indicating lack of coordination between respiration and phonation.

Eyes

Look for nystagmus by asking him to look straight ahead while you hold his forehead with your left hand. Hold your right index finger about 50 cm in front of his eyes and ask the patient to follow your finger with his eyes while you move your finger from one side to the other in the mid-horizontal plane. See if there is any nystagmus at the right and left extremes of his gaze. Do not take your finger too far laterally on either side because extreme abduction of the eyes can cause nystagmus even in normal eyes.

Arms

Coordination in the arms can be demonstrated by pronating and supinating the forearms as rapidly as possible with the elbows at a right angle. Ask the patient next to approximate the fingertips of both hands and then rapidly separate them and bring them back together repeatedly (Fig. 4.6.1). You can also ask the patient to tap quickly on the back of his hand and to alternate tapping with the palmar and the dorsal surface of the fingers — this can accentuate even mild incoordination. (Impairment of rapid alternate movements is known as *dysdiadochokinesis*.) Lastly, perform the *finger–nose test*. Hold out your right index finger and ask the patient to touch your finger with his index finger, then to touch the tip of his nose, doing this backwards and forwards quickly and neatly. (Demonstrate if necessary and vary the target.) Ask him to repeat this with his other hand. Look for *past-pointing* and an *intention tremor* (increases on approaching the target).

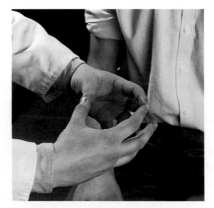

Fig. 4.6.1 Testing coordination

Legs

Again, test coordination by asking the patient to perform the *heel–shin test*. Explain to the patient what you intend to do and test, and then lift his right heel and leave it in the air above his left knee (Fig. 4.6.2). Ask him to place his right heel on his left knee and run it smoothly up and down the left shin (Fig. 4.6.3). Ask him to do this a few times and then to repeat the manoeuvre with his other heel. Watch for any clumsiness while he attempts to accomplish this task. He may not be able to keep his heel on the shin all the way down. Then ask him to tap on your hand with his foot (Fig. 4.6.4).

Gait

Ask the patient if he can walk unaided. If he reports some difficulty then reassure him that you will stay with him in case of

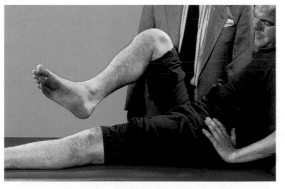

Fig. 4.6.2 Starting the heel–shin test

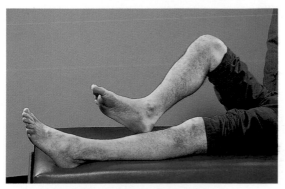

Fig. 4.6.3 Running along the shin

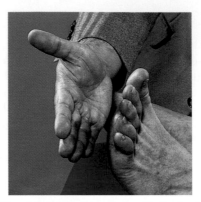

Fig. 4.6.4 Quick tapping with the foot

any problems. Ask him to walk towards a defined point and back while you look for signs of a wide-based *ataxic gait*, noting also any clumsiness at the turn. Next, demonstrate and test heel-to-toe walking (see Fig. 4.5.6; p. 282), which will exacerbate ataxia. (Note the side to which the patient tends to fall.)

While you were examining the patient you may have noticed other useful signs which could give you clues about underlying causes for a cerebellar syndrome such as *internuclear ophthalmoplegia* (demyelination), *clubbing* (malignancy), or *pes cavus* (Friedreich's ataxia), and you can mention these in your presentation. However, your conclusion must address principally the integrity of the cerebellar system and should include comments on the articulation of speech, the presence or absence of nystagmus, and on whether the patient has ataxia when his eyes are open.

This is Mr Rowe. I would like you to examine his second to seventh cranial nerves explaining each step as you go through the examination.

The purpose of this station is not only to test your examination skills but also to see if you can develop a good rapport with the patient, and how you enlist his cooperation and explain the essentials of the examination (to both the examiner and the patient). Summarize what you are going to do at each major step to the examiner before explaining each component to the patient. After examining each cranial nerve, present your findings to the examiner. When you have finished, summarize the outcome of the entire examination first to the examiner and then, in simple language, to the patient.

To the patient: Hello, Mr Rowe. Good morning. I am Dr Singh and I have been asked to examine your eyes and face. I hope you don't mind. (*Pause*) I will explain everything as I go along but if there is anything you do not understand or wish to ask please do not hesitate to stop me.

To the examiner: I will start by looking at the patient's face for *ptosis*, suggestive of myasthenia gravis, a third nerve palsy, or Horner's syndrome; *unequal pupils*, suggestive of a myotonic pupil, a third nerve palsy or Horner's; and for *facial asymmetry*, suggestive of a fifth or seventh nerve palsy. (*Look at the patient's face and make a comment on whether its appearance is normal.*)
    I will now test the *second cranial nerve* whose functions include conduction of the afferent impulses for the light reflex, for which I'll use a torch, and vision. I'll test visual acuity with a portable Snellen's chart (Fig. 4.7.1); near vision with a booklet of small prints (Fig. 4.7.2); colour vision with the Ishihara chart (Fig. 4.7.3); central vision with a red hatpin; the visual fields by

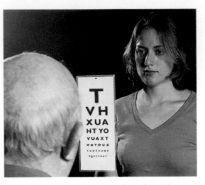

Fig. 4.7.1 Testing visual acuity

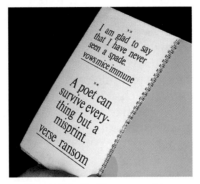

Fig. 4.7.2 Testing near vision

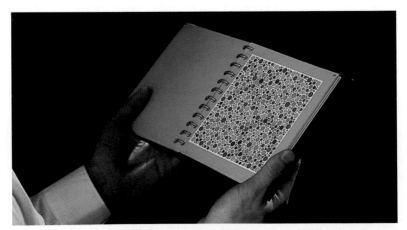

Fig. 4.7.3 Testing colour vision

confrontation against mine; and the fundi with an
ophthalmoscope.

*If this equipment is not available you can test the visual acuity by
asking the patient to read the time on the clock on the wall. Make sure
he is wearing his glasses if he uses them for distant vision, or use a
pinhole. You can test colour vision with your red and white hatpins,
and the near vision by asking him to read a passage in a book or a
newspaper.*

To the patient: Mr Rowe, I am going to shine my torch on your
eyes to test the reaction of your pupils. It has a strong beam
(*make sure it has!*) but I won't shine it for long. Now, if you
would look at the wall while I shine it (Fig. 4.7.4). (*Make sure
you examine both pupils for the direct and consensual reflexes.*)
  Now I would like to test your eyesight by asking you to read
this card while I hold it up here (Fig. 4.7.1). One eye at a time,
so please close your right eye first, but keep your glasses on and
see if you can read to the last line. Now let us try the other eye.
That is fine, thank you.
  I would now like to test your near vision. I'll hold this book
(*about 30 cm from his eyes*) and you show me the smallest print you
can read (Fig. 4.7.2). Yes, that is fine, thank you. Now, can you
show me a cross and a circle on this Ishihara chart (Fig. 4.7.3)?
That is very good.
  You are doing very well, Mr Rowe. I am now going to test your
field of vision against mine, while I sit about a metre away from
you. I'll test one eye at a time while we close our opposing eyes,

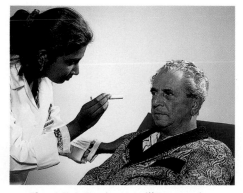

Fig. 4.7.4 Testing pupillary reaction

that is your left eye and my right eye, like this (*demonstrate*). I'll bring my index finger in from the side slowly — please tell me as soon as you can see it. (*Test other parts of the visual field on this side.*) You can now close your right eye and I will close my left eye while I bring my right index finger in (Fig. 4.7.5). (*Again, test other segments of the visual field on this side.*)

While we are sitting like this I will try the same exercise with my red-headed hatpin — you keep looking at it and tell me as soon as either the head disappears or it changes colour (Fig. 4.7.6). That is very good. Thank you very much. Now I would like to look in your eyes with this special torch while you try to look as far into the distance as possible.

Summarize your findings to the examiner and explain the next set of steps to him.

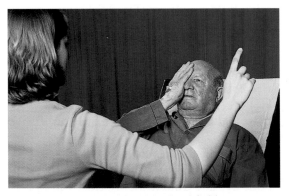

Fig. 4.7.5 Testing visual fields

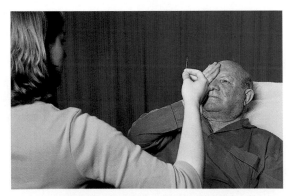

Fig. 4.7.6 Testing central vision

To the examiner: I will now test the *third, fourth, and sixth cranial nerves* by asking the patient to follow my moving finger. I'll take it first to the right, then up and down, and then to the left and again up and down in the shape of an 'H'.

To the patient: Please look at my finger and follow it wherever it goes, while I keep your head still with my left hand (Fig. 4.7.7). As I move my finger you may see two fingers. If you do, please tell me which is the false image and what it looks like. That is fine, thank you. (*Summarize your findings to the examiner.*)

To the examiner: Finally, I am going to test the *fifth and seventh cranial nerves* by testing facial movements and sensations.

To the patient: Mr Rowe, we are coming to the end of this examination. Thank you for being so patient. I am going to ask you to perform certain movements and now and again I might resist them, just to test your strength. I won't hurt you. (*For each manoeuvre demonstrate what you would like him to do.*)

Now, please raise your eyebrows, as I am doing. Screw up your eyes (Fig. 4.7.8). That is fine. Now, puff your cheeks out, like this.

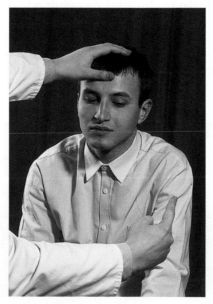

Fig. 4.7.7 Testing eye movements

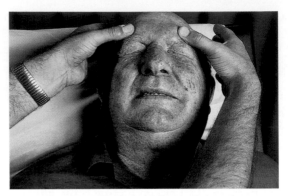

Fig. 4.7.8 Testing the frontalis muscles

Whistle. Show me your teeth. Now clench them. (*Feel the masseters* (Fig. 4.7.9) *and temporalis.*) Now open your mouth and stop me closing it.

Now I am going to test whether you can feel this cotton wool on your face while you keep your eyes closed. Please say 'yes' whenever you feel my touch. I will say nothing — I'll just touch, and you say 'yes' when you feel it (*demonstrate*). While you keep your eyes closed I'll touch you with either a piece of cotton wool or a paper clip, and you must tell me what I am touching you with. Do you understand? Fine. Here we go. (*After testing sensation, test the corneal reflex.*) As you look at my eyes, I will dab this cotton wisp onto your eyeball to see your reaction (Fig. 4.7.10). This is the last bit — it will be quick and I won't

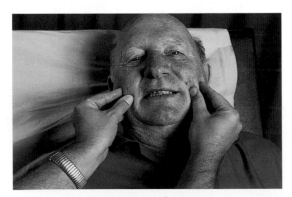

Fig. 4.7.9 Testing the masseters

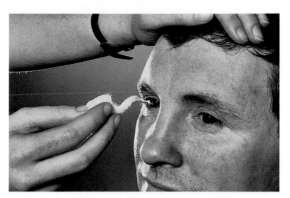

Fig. 4.7.10 Testing the corneal reflex

hurt you. You just keep looking straight ahead while I dab this wisp quickly. Are you ready? Fine, thank you.

Summarize your findings and diagnosis to the examiner, then explain to the patient and thank him.

Please examine this patient's fundi.

There may be a couple of surprises waiting for you at this station. First, you may find that it is not a real patient but a manikin. This should not unsettle you and you should treat the manikin in the same way as you would a patient. Introduce yourself to the patient, real or manikin, and explain that you have been asked to examine the back of the eyes: that you will look at the front of the eyes first; then shine a light onto each eye in turn; and finally, look through the ophthalmoscope:

To the patient: The light is not too strong but you may find it a little uncomfortable. Please try to relax and look into the distance as if you are trying to see an aeroplane in the sky. I'll try to be as brief as possible, but I have to look at the back of the eye and it may take a minute or so on each side. Would that be all right?

Explain to the examiner that you would first have a general look at the patient for any obvious signs of disease, such as diabetes mellitus (necrobiosis lipoidica, foot ulcers). You would look at the eyes and note whether there is *arcus lipidus*, which, in a younger patient (rare), would suggest diabetes mellitus. You would then stand about a half a metre away from the patient and look through the ophthalmoscope shining the light on each eye in turn. Tell the examiner that you are looking for the *red reflex* of the retina, which can be seen if the media from the cornea to the retina are clear and there is no cataract. (You have to mention this because there will be no red reflex in a manikin!) Now move in towards the patient's right eye and look at it with your right eye, using the plus dioptre lenses to focus on the structures in front of the retina. As you go down the lenses you will see the lens, the vitreous, and finally the retina. You will be looking for opacities, haemorrhages, or new vessels in the vitreous.

At this stage you may get your second surprise. Just as you thought that you had gone through all the motions and had finished your examination, the examiner might project a colour slide of a fundus for you to describe and diagnose! This should not cause you any problems because these pictures are generally easier to see than the limited view through an ophthalmoscope. You should familiarize yourself with the appearances of some common conditions before the exam.

Diabetic retinopathy

There may be *background retinopathy* with *microaneurysms*, and dot and blot *retinal haemorrhages* (Fig. 4.8.1). There may be more advanced changes with *hard exudates*, which have well-defined margins (Fig. 4.8.2). These represent the lipid remains of vascular leakage and may be distributed in a circle round a vascular abnormality (circinate exudate). The term *maculopathy* is applied to the condition when the haemorrhages or exudates are either on or around the macula (Fig. 4.8.3). A patient with this condition should be referred to an ophthalmologist. Fluffy *soft exudates* (cotton wool spots) with indistinct margins, hard exudates and margins may herald the onset of preproliferative

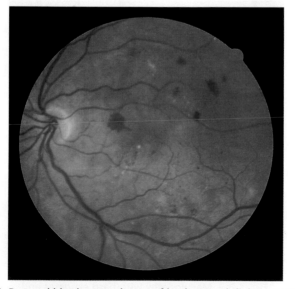

Fig. 4.8.1 Dot and blot haemorrhages of background diabetic retinopathy

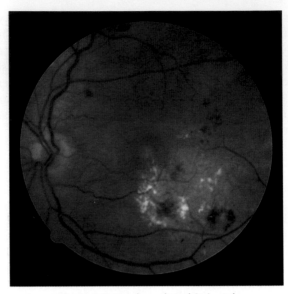

Fig. 4.8.2 Hard exudate (circinate)

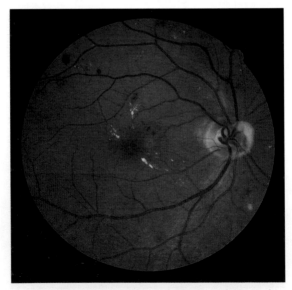

Fig. 4.8.3 Maculopathy with hard exudates and haemorrhages around the macula

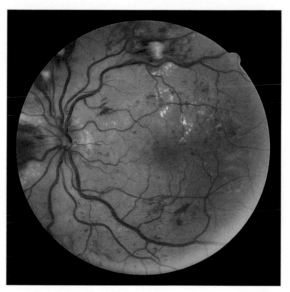

Fig. 4.8.4 Haemorrhages and hard and soft exudates

retinopathy (Fig. 4.8.4). *Neovascularization* may be seen, with sheaths of new vessels sprouting from the retina, often with haemorrhages and exudates — *proliferative retinopathy*.

Hypertensive retinopathy

This may be of any severity, ranging from *grade 1* to frank *papilloedema (grade 4)*. In grade 1 hypertensive retinopathy there is *reactive sclerosis*, when the vessels become narrower and straighter with a reduced axial reflex, and the arteries become paler and branch more acutely. In grade 2 hypertensive retinopathy there is, in addition to these changes, *arteriovenous nipping*. In grade 3 hypertensive retinopathy you will often see soft and hard exudates and *flame-shaped haemorrhages* (Fig. 4.8.5).

Papilloedema

Papilloedema (Fig. 4.8.6) is a cardinal feature of accelerated hypertension (grade 4 hypertensive retinopathy) but it is also caused by raised intracranial pressure. The disc margins become oedematous and blurred, and the veins in the surrounding retina

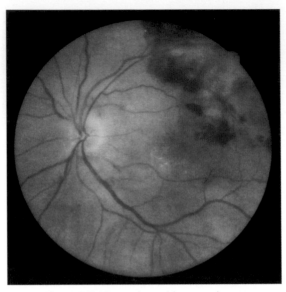

Fig. 4.8.5 Flame-shaped haemorrhages

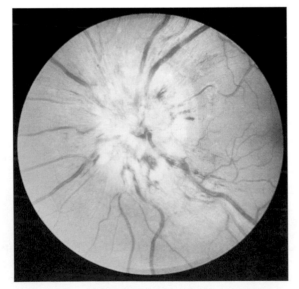

Fig. 4.8.6 Papilloedema

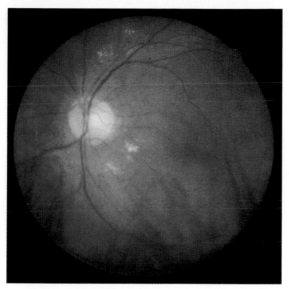

Fig. 4.8.7 Pale disc with attenuated vessels

tortuous and dilated. There are hard exudates and fluffy haemorrhages when hypertension is the underlying cause of papilloedema.

Optic atrophy

Primary optic atrophy may result from compression, toxic, or ischaemic damage to the optic nerve. The disc is excessively pale, with sharply defined margins and the retinal vessels appear attenuated (Fig. 4.8.7).

Choroidoretinitis

A variety of microbial infections (bacteria, fungi, protozoa, viruses, rickettsia) and systemic disorders (sarcoidosis, onchocerciasis) may affect the choroid and retina. In chronic cases there is pigmentation surrounding an area of necrosis of the choroid and retina (Fig. 4.8.8). Cytomegalovirus infection of the retina typically occurs in patients with AIDS. In this condition there is retinitis without choroiditis, producing a whitish patch streaked with haemorrhages which has been likened to the appearance of scrambled egg with tomato sauce.

299

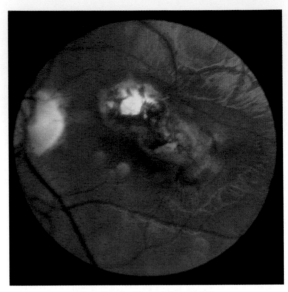

Fig. 4.8.8 Choroidoretinitis

Please examine this patient's visual fields.

The patient to be examined may be a healthy volunteer and the examiner's purpose will be to scrutinize how you test the visual fields; on the other hand, there may be a real patient with a field defect.

After the initial introductory remarks and explanations to the patient, ask the patient to sit upright on the side of the couch while you look for any signs that might be associated with a field defect (e.g. hemiparesis with a *homonymous hemianopia* or acromegaly with *bitemporal or unilateral hemianopia*, or *quadrantic field defects*).

Ensure that the patient can see with both eyes — *do not mistake a visual acuity problem for a field defect.* You could ask the patient whether his vision is normal or ask him to read the time (with each eye in turn) on a clock on the wall. However, it is better to adopt a more professional approach and use a portable Snellen's chart (see Fig. 4.7.1; p. 288). Stand about 2 metres in front of the patient and ask him to read the lines on the card with each eye in turn.

Now sit in front of the patient, about a metre away, and ask him to look at your eyes while you place your index fingers just inside the outer limits of your own temporal fields. Move your fingers one at a time and then both at the same time (Fig. 4.9.1) and ask the patient to point to the moving finger or fingers. If he has *visual inattention*, he will point to only one finger when you are moving *both*. (Make sure that he can see both fingers individually but only one when they are moving both together.)

Next, test each eye individually against your opposing eye (see Fig. 4.7.5; p. 290). Ask him to close his right eye with his right index finger while you close your left eye. Explain and demonstrate this to him and ask him to keep looking with his

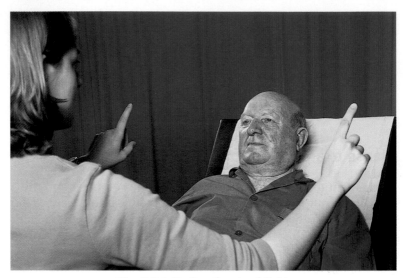

Fig. 4.9.1 Testing the visual fields

left eye at your right eye, which you will keep fixed on his. Move your wagging finger in slowly and ask him to tell you as soon as he sees your finger move. After bringing your finger in horizontally you should repeat the procedure, moving in from the upper and lower temporal quadrants. This tests his left temporal vision against your right temporal field. To test the nasal field of his left eye against the nasal field of your right eye, move your left index finger in from just outside the limit of your own nasal field (Fig. 4.9.2). Repeat this procedure on his right eye, comparing its visual fields to those of your left eye. This comparison of the patient's visual fields against yours should enable you to map out any defects.

Next, you should test the patient's central vision, unless the examiner stops you. To test his left eye against your right eye use a red-headed hatpin and bring it in horizontally from the temporal periphery, through the central field, to the nasal periphery. (Fig. 4.9.3). Ask him to tell you as soon as he sees the head of the pin. Then ask him to keep looking at it and tell you if it disappears or changes colour from red to white. Compare his blind spot with your own and note if his blind spot is enlarged or if there is an additional defect (*scotoma*).

Summarize your findings to the examiner.

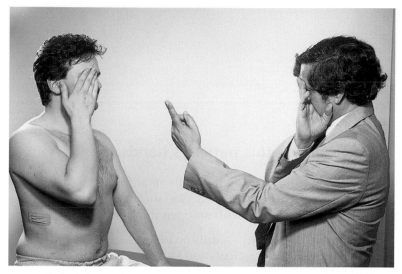

Fig. 4.9.2 Testing the left nasal field

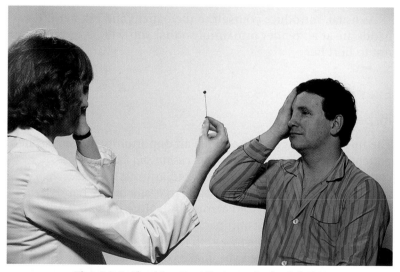

Fig. 4.9.3 Checking the blind spot in the left eye

Please examine this patient's hands.

This station usually has a patient with an arthropathy (e.g. rheumatoid, osteoarthrosis, gout, psoriatic arthropathy) but you should approach the task with an open mind, looking for:

- Swelling and deformity — arthropathy
- Wasting, deformity, fasciculation — neuromuscular disorders
- Skin rash, clubbing, xanthomata — dermatoses, systemic disorders

As usual, introduce yourself to the patient and ask her if her hands are at all tender or painful so that you will be extra careful not to hurt her.

Examination

Inspection

The initial exchanges will provide an opportunity to look at the patient's face to see if she appears *cushingoid* (e.g. due to corticosteroid therapy for rheumatoid arthritis), *acromegalic* (prominent supraorbital ridge and large, spade-like hands), or has exophthalmos (thyroid acropachy). Note if she has adherent shiny skin over the face and neck, with or without telangiectasia (associated with *sclerodactyly*, with tapering of the fingers, in systemic sclerosis). When you make your presentation remember to include any of these general observations in support of your diagnosis. You would mention, for example, hairline psoriasis plaques in a patient with psoriatic arthropathy.

Inspect the hands to decide whether the patient has an arthropathy, a neuromuscular disorder, or a cutaneous condition. You may be able to develop a diagnostic impression about one of the conditions that is usually presented in this examination.

Arthropathy

There may be proximal joint swelling, spindling of the fingers, ulnar deviation, and nodules in rheumatoid arthritis (Fig. 4.10.1); Heberden's nodes, sometimes with flexion or lateral deformity of the terminal phalanges, bony enlargements, or subluxation of the first metacarpophalangeal joints, producing the square-hand deformity of osteoarthrosis (Fig. 4.10.2); or tophaceous deposits with joint deformities in gout (Fig. 4.10.3).

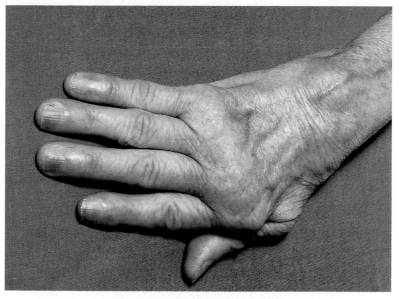

Fig. 4.10.1 Rheumatoid arthritis

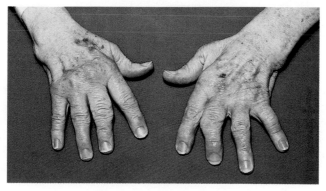

Fig. 4.10.2 Osteoarthrosis

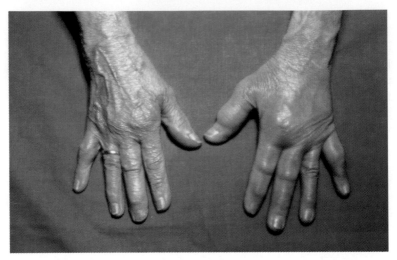

Fig. 4.10.3 Gout

Neuromuscular disorders

There may be generalized wasting of the small muscles of the hand, with dorsal guttering and fasciculation in motor neurone disease (Fig. 4.10.4); a claw hand in ulnar nerve palsy (Fig. 4.10.5); and isolated wasting of the thenar eminence (rare these days) in carpal tunnel syndrome (Fig. 4.10.6).

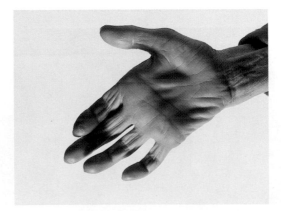

Fig. 4.10.4 Wasting of the small muscles of the hand

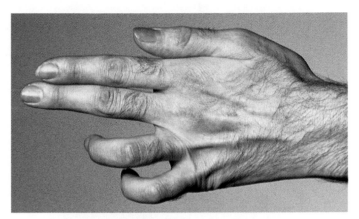

Fig. 4.10.5 Ulnar nerve palsy — claw hand

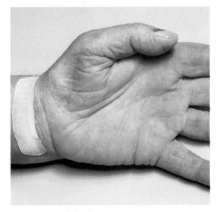

Fig. 4.10.6 Thenar wasting

Cutaneous conditions

You may see pitting of the nails, terminal interphalangeal arthropathy (Fig. 4.10.7), and a scaly rash on the extensor surfaces of the extremities in psoriasis.

Palpation

Arthropathy

If there is an arthropathy you should note carefully which joints are swollen or deformed and proceed to palpate the hands *gently*. Take extra care not to hurt the patient. Remember to look at the elbows for any rheumatoid nodules or patches of psoriasis. Test movements of the joints of the hand by asking

307

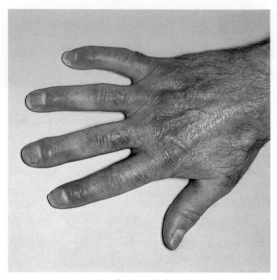

Fig. 4.10.7 Terminal interphalangeal arthropathy

the patient to make a fist. Demonstrate, and then check wrist extension (Fig. 4.10.8) and flexion (Fig. 4.10.9). Note the extent of limitation of movements. Next, assess function by asking the patient how much she can do with her hands. For example, can she use a knife and fork? If there is a severe degree of deformity you may ask the patient whether she can pick up a paper clip with the fingers of one hand.

Give a complete summary of your findings, with the diagnosis, to the examiner. For example:

> This lady has a bilateral deforming arthropathy with swelling of the metacarpophalangeal and proximal interphalangeal joints; muscle wasting and subluxation of the metacarpophalangeal joints resulting in ulnar deviation; and nodules on the right elbow. All the movements in the hands are limited but she has retained a reasonable degree of function and manoeuvrability. The diagnosis is moderately severe rheumatoid arthritis.

Neuromuscular disorders

If you suspect a neuromuscular disorder you should note the findings on inspection and carry out a neurological examination. Check the tone of the muscles in the hand by flexing and

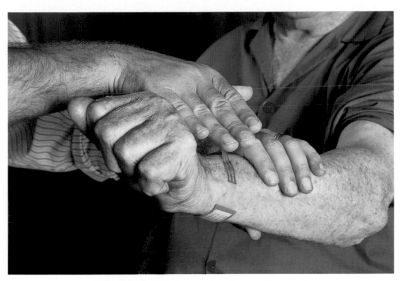

Fig. 4.10.8 Testing extension at the wrist

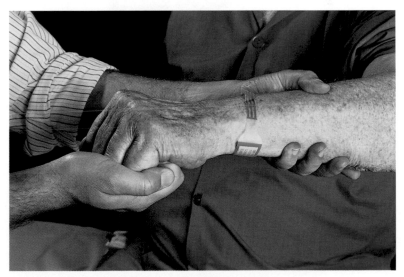

Fig. 4.10.9 Testing flexion at the wrist

extending all the joints including the wrist in a 'rolling wave' fashion. Test the motor system of the hands by making a series of requests:

- *C8, T1.* Squeeze my fingers (Fig. 4.10.10).
- *C7, radial nerve.* Hold your fingers straight and stop me pressing them down (Fig. 4.10.11).
- *Dorsal interossei, ulnar nerve.* Hold your fingers apart and stop me pressing them together (Fig. 4.10.12). (Remember, DAB = dorsal abduct.)
- *Palmar interossei, ulnar nerve.* Hold this piece of paper between your fingers and try to stop me pulling it out (Fig. 4.10.13). (Remember, PAD = palmar adduct.)

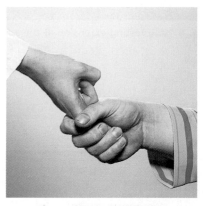

Fig. 4.10.10 Testing grip

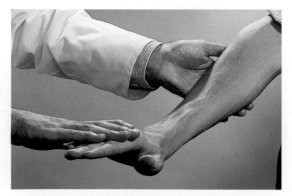

Fig. 4.10.11 Testing extension of the fingers

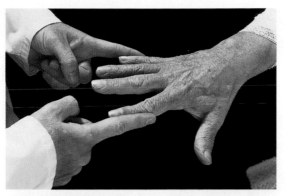

Fig. 4.10.12 Testing abduction of the fingers

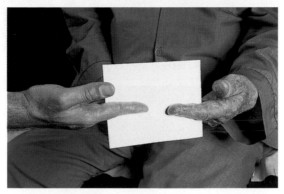

Fig. 4.10.13 Testing adduction of the fingers

- *Abductor pollicis brevis, median nerve.* Point your thumb at the ceiling; stop me pushing it down (Fig. 4.10.14).
- *Opponens pollicis, median nerve.* Put your thumb and little finger together; stop me pulling them apart.

Complete the examination by checking *sensation*, first for light touch (dab cotton wool lightly); then for pinprick, using a paper clip or a disposable pin (Fig. 4.10.15); and then for vibration and joint position sense. Define any area of deficit to see if it corresponds to ulnar or median nerve sensory distribution (Fig. 4.10.16). Ask the patient if there has been any numbness or tingling in the hands and, if so, when (this tends to be worse at night in carpal tunnel syndrome).

Thank the patient and give a complete description of your findings and diagnosis to the examiner.

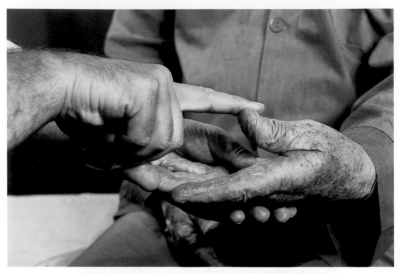

Fig. 4.10.14 Testing abductor pollicis brevis

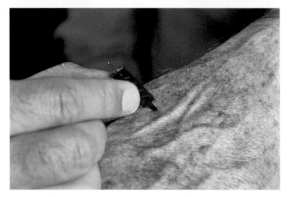

Fig. 4.10.15 Testing pinprick sensation

Cutaneous conditions

If the object of the exercise is to test your expertise in dermatology it is likely to be a common condition, with which you are familiar (e.g. psoriasis, vitiligo, drug rash, etc.). Study an individual lesion and decide whether it is a macule, papule, plaque, nodule, or a vesicle; look for secondary phenomena (scratch marks, crusts, scars, scales or lichenification); and examine its distribution. Even if you cannot make an accurate diagnosis you should be able to give a good description, with appropriate terminology.

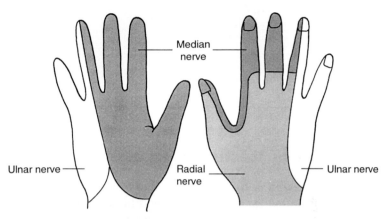

Fig. 4.10.16 Sensory distribution of median, radial, and ulnar nerves

For the sake of completeness, and specifically if there is any vascular disturbance (cyanosis, ulcers on the fingertips, pallor), you should check the radial pulses in both wrists. You should also be alert to clues elsewhere on the body, such as osteoarthrosis in the elbow or a scar over the elbow in ulnar nerve palsy, tophi on the ears in gout, or signs of acromegaly or hypothyroidism in association with carpal tunnel syndrome.

Please examine the arterial pulses of this patient.

You will be assessed in three main areas in this station. First, the examiner will watch carefully to see if you have acquired the appropriate skills for examining the principal pulses (radial, brachial and carotid) and whether you are able to interpret the information so gained. Secondly, whether the subject is a real patient with some abnormality, a volunteer, or a manikin, the examiner will be assessing whether you can locate all the accessible pulses and palpate them properly. As you have been asked to examine 'the arterial pulses', you will have to extend your examination beyond the upper torso and demonstrate your competence at palpating the femoral, popliteal, posterior tibial and dorsalis pedis pulses (Fig. 4.11.1). Thirdly, if there is an abnormality you will be expected to identify and describe it. You should bear the following abnormalities in mind even if the subject is a manikin:

- Bradycardia (<60 beats per minute)
- Tachycardia (>90 beats per minute)
- Irregular pulse (e.g. ectopics, atrial fibrillation)
- Collapsing pulse (aortic incompetence, patent ductus arteriosus, large arteriovenous fistula)
- Small-volume pulse (aortic stenosis, mitral stenosis)
- Absent pulse (thromboembolism, peripheral vascular disease)
- Complete heart block
- Radiofemoral delay (coarctation of the aorta)
- Pulsus paradoxus (rare in this exam)

Examination

Inspection

As always, start with the patient's face and look for any malar flush (mitral stenosis), for any signs of hypothyroidism

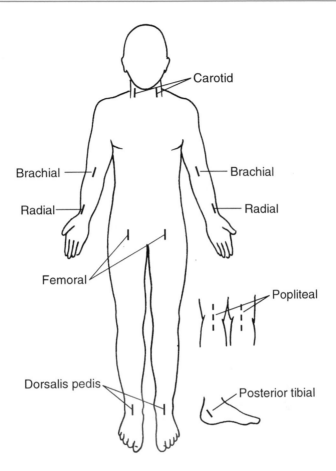

Fig. 4.11.1 Accessible pulses

(thickened and coarse facial features, sparse and brittle eyebrows, pallor), or of hyperthyroidism (exophthalmos, lid lag). Look at the neck for raised jugular venous pressure, Corrigan's sign (a large upstroke of the carotid pulse and an abrupt fall), goitre or a thyroidectomy scar. Run your eyes over the chest (pulsations, scars), abdomen (ascites), hands (cyanosis, clubbing), and legs (oedema, cyanosis, ulcers, gangrene). This survey should be carried out while you feel the right radial pulse.

315

Palpation

Feel the patient's right radial pulse with the middle three fingers of your hand and note its *rate* (count for 15 seconds) and *rhythm*, whether it is regular or irregular (check pause-to-pause variability). Palpate the upstroke of the pulse wave with the pulp of your finger to appreciate the *volume*, whether it is large-volume (diastolic overload) or slow-rising (aortic stenosis). You will be able to gain an initial impression of the *character* (pulse wave) which you can confirm later by feeling the brachial and carotid pulses. Using the scheme outlined below should ensure that you miss nothing important.

1. If the pulse has a large volume then you should check whether it has a *collapsing*, or *water-hammer*, character, by placing the palm of one hand over the patient's wrist and the palm of the other over the axillary artery and then lifting the patient's hand above his head (see Fig. 4.1.1; p. 251). If the pulse has a collapsing character you will feel a sharp flick (a sharp upstroke and an abrupt fall) across both your palms. This is characteristic of haemodynamically significant aortic incompetence and patent ductus arteriosus.
2. If the upstroke is small or flat then you can assess whether it is a *slow-rising* or *plateau* pulse by palpating the brachial artery with the pulp of your thumb (Fig. 4.11.2). As you press (gently) you may feel the *anacrotic notch* on the upstroke

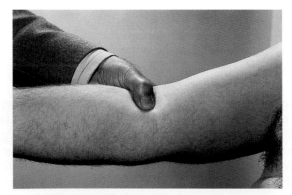

Fig. 4.11.2 Feeling the brachial pulse

against the pulp of your thumb. In mixed aortic valve disease the combination of plateau and collapsing effects can produce a double-peaked *pulsus bisferiens*.

3. Feel the opposite radial pulse to see if it is present and of equal volume. It may be absent either because of a proximal thromboembolism or because a Blalock shunt has been performed as a palliative procedure for Fallot's tetralogy. A feeble pulse on either side may be caused by atherosclerosis.

4. Next, feel the right carotid pulse with your left thumb, where you can appreciate the character of the pulse (see Fig. 4.1.2; p. 251), whether slow-rising, or collapsing with a large upstroke and an abrupt fall (*Corrigan's sign*). Feel the opposite carotid to determine whether it is present and of equal volume. If one carotid pulse is absent or feeble you must listen over it for a bruit later.

5. Feel the right femoral pulse and note if there is any *radiofemoral delay* suggestive of coarctation of the aorta. Feel the opposite femoral (Fig. 4.1.3) and note if they are equal in volume.

6. With the knee joint semiflexed, feel the popliteal artery with both hands, first on the right side and then on the left side. If you experience any difficulty ask the patient to lie on his front, as the popliteal pulse may be easier to feel in a prone subject (Fig. 4.11.3). Next, feel the posterior tibial (Fig. 4.11.4) and the dorsalis pedis (Fig. 4.11.5) pulses on both sides.

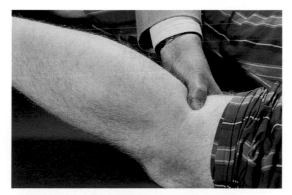

Fig. 4.11.3 Feeling the popliteal pulse

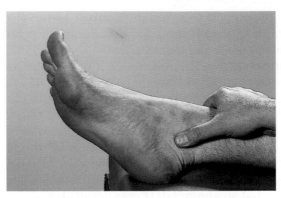

Fig. 4.11.4 Feeling the posterior tibial pulse

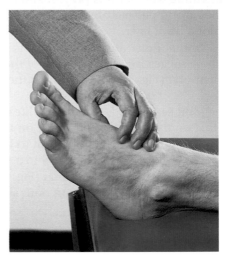

Fig. 4.11.5 Feeling the dorsalis pedis pulse

Auscultation

You should listen over the carotids and femorals for *bruits*, particularly if any of the pulses are absent or reduced in volume.

Please examine this patient's lymph glands.

The examiner will have three objectives in assessing you at this station. First, she will want to know whether you have an orthodox examination technique and are familiar with it. For example, approaching the lymph glands of the neck from the front of the patient will instantly bring you to the pass/fail borderline. Second, she wants you to demonstrate your knowledge of where the glands are situated, and that you can examine them sequentially and methodically while you keep the subject at ease. Third, if and when you do find an enlarged gland, she will be observing whether you correctly apply the principles of examination of a swelling. You should rehearse the various steps of this examination on a friend, colleague, or volunteer so that your technique becomes slick and professional.

Briefly introduce yourself to the patient and explain the purpose of the examination and what it will entail. Ask him to tell you if any of the regions you will be examining is tender or painful. Reassure him that you will be gentle and reasonably quick.

Examination

Cervical nodes

Sit the patient in a chair or on the edge of a couch and approach from behind to examine the glands in the neck. Feel in the anterior and posterior triangles of the neck with one hand, while using the other hand to flex the patient's neck slightly (Fig. 4.12.1). Push your finger gently behind the medial end of the clavicle to feel for an enlarged scalene node. After palpating the neck on both sides, feel the undersurface of the chin for submental nodes, below the angle of the jaw for tonsillar nodes, in front of and behind the ear for pre- and postauricular nodes, and below the hairline posteriorly for suboccipital nodes.

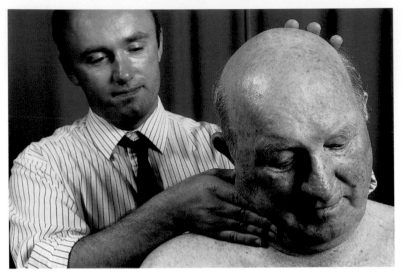

Fig. 4.12.1 Palpating the cervical lymph nodes

Axillary nodes

You can examine the axillary lymph glands either with the patient lying supine or sitting up facing you with his left arm resting on your palpating right wrist (Fig. 4.12.2). Work your

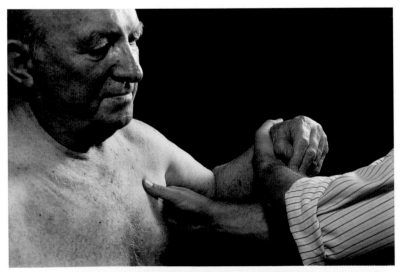

Fig. 4.12.2 Palpating axillary lymph nodes

fingers gently upwards to palpate the apex and the medial wall of the axilla. Repeat this procedure on the patient's right axilla with your left hand. Then examine the sitting patient from behind to feel the subscapular glands along the posterior axillary fold.

Epitrochlear nodes

These nodes, when enlarged, can be felt just proximal to the medial epicondyle with the patient's elbow semiflexed and his hand resting on your opposite hand.

Inguinal nodes

The subject should be lying supine with the inguinal regions exposed. Feel above the inguinal ligament for the superior inguinal nodes, below it for the inferior inguinal nodes, and vertically for the longitudinal group of lymph nodes along the femoral vessels. Repeat the procedure on the opposite side.

If you feel a swelling, note its *shape* and *consistency* (hard and craggy in metastatic disease, firm and rubbery in lymphoma), measure its *dimensions*, and determine whether it is *freely mobile* or *fixed to deep structures* (see p. 339). Make sure that you do not miss any lesion that may be the cause of the enlarged glands.

Please examine this patient's thyroid gland.

The patient may have an easily visible goitre; he may have only a modest enlargement of the thyroid gland; or he may be a healthy volunteer with a normal, scarcely visible gland. The examiner will be assessing whether you can perform a competent examination. There may be a glass of water purposely left on the table by the side of the patient. Thank the examiner and introduce yourself to the patient, explaining what you intend to do.

Examination

Inspection

Position yourself at the right side of the patient and look at the neck for any swelling of the thyroid gland, any discoloration of the overlying skin, and for any scars. Offer the patient the glass of water. Ask him to take a sip, hold it in his mouth, and then swallow it, while you observe his neck. As the patient swallows the sip of water the whole gland will move upwards, giving you some idea of its size and shape. A nodule hitherto invisible behind the sternomastoid muscle may become visible.

Palpation

Stand behind the right side of the patient so that you can feel, as well as see, the gland when you ask him to swallow another sip of water during palpation. Slightly flex the neck with your left hand and place your index finger below the cricoid cartilage, where the isthmus of the thyroid gland lies over the trachea (Fig. 4.13.1). Gently extend the palpation laterally (Fig. 4.13.2) to feel the two lobes of the thyroid gland, which lie behind the sternomastoid muscle. Ask the patient to swallow again while you continue to palpate. Extend palpation along the medial

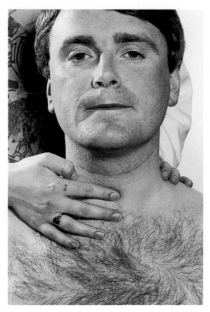

Fig. 4.13.1 Feeling for the isthmus of the thyroid

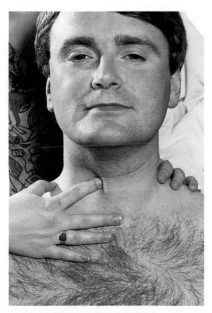

Fig. 4.13.2 Feeling for the right lobe of the thyroid

323

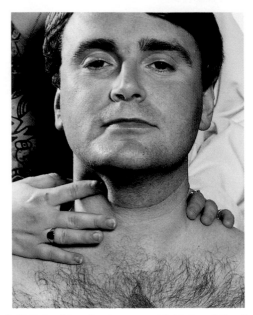

Fig. 4.13.3 Looking for the pyramidal lobe of the thyroid

border of the sternomastoid muscles on both sides to look for the presence of a pyramidal lobe (Fig. 4.13.3). Watch the patient's face for signs of any discomfort that you may cause during deep palpation as the thyroid gland, particularly in Graves' disease and subacute thyroiditis, can be tender. Apologize to the patient and reassure him that you are nearly finished.

If the thyroid gland is enlarged you should make a note of its size; whether it is soft or firm; whether it is nodular or diffusely enlarged; whether it moves freely on swallowing or is tethered to the underlying structures or the skin; whether the overlying skin is discolored; whether there are lymph nodes; and whether there is a vascular murmur audible over it. You will need all this information for your presentation.

Palpate the rest of the neck to feel for any lymph nodes. If there is a goitre you could percuss gently over the manubrium, where a dull note may suggest a retrosternal extension.

Auscultation

Listen over the thyroid (with the diaphragm) for evidence of increased vascularity in Graves' disease. If you hear a systolic bruit you should rule out the presence of a venous hum by occluding the venous return, and also listen over the aortic area to avoid confusion with a conducted murmur.

Thank the patient and apologize once again for any discomfort you may have caused.

Please examine this patient's thyroid status.

You are being asked here to assess whether the patient is clinically hyperthyroid, euthyroid, or hypothyroid. The patient may show *signs* of thyroid disease (exophthalmos, goitre, etc.) but you are not expected to explore these, only note their presence during your initial observation. The presence of a goitre, thyroid acropachy, pretibial myxoedema, or the typical facial characteristics of myxoedema may provide useful clues. Observe the patient's demeanour, whether she is hyperactive and fidgety (hyperthyroid), or somewhat immobile and uninterested in her surroundings (hypothyroid).

Take the radial *pulse* (count for 15 seconds), noting the presence or absence of atrial fibrillation (slow, normal rate, or fast). If the pulse is slow (less than 60 beats per minute) or if you suspect hypothyroidism from the patient's appearance, go on to test the *ankle reflexes* looking for the typical *slow relaxation* (demonstrated best at the ankle but also found in the supinator and other reflexes). When testing the reflexes (see p. 281) you need to enlist the patient's cooperation and as you chat with her about what you are doing, you will not only put her at ease, but may also spot more helpful clues (e.g. slow, hesitant speech, sluggish movements). If you experience difficulty obtaining the ankle jerk, get the patient to kneel on a chair (Fig. 4.14.1). If the pulse is normal or fast, feel the patient's *palms* (warm and sweaty in hyperthyroidism; cold and sweaty in anxiety) and ask the patient to stretch out her hands, wrists and elbows fully extended. If a *tremor* is not obvious place a piece of paper on the outstretched hands — it will shake if a fine tremor is present.

Look at the eyes noting exophthalmos (in which sclera is visible above the lower lid, but a sign not always related to thyroid disease) and look especially for *lid retraction* (in which sclera is visible *above* the cornea). Test for *lid lag* by asking the

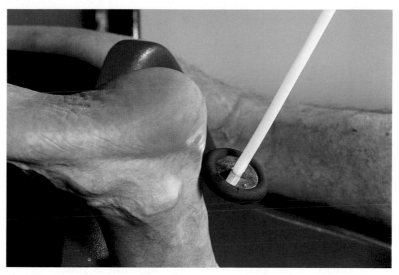

Fig. 4.14.1 Testing the ankle reflex

patient to follow your moving finger with her eyes, from above downwards. Your finger should be about 18 cm away and you should complete the movement from above downwards in 2 seconds. In Graves' disease, the upper lids will lag behind the downward movement of the eyeballs.

Examine the neck if there is a goitre present, remembering the steps (look, palpate, and auscultate). A *thyroid bruit* is good evidence of hyperthyroidism.

Putting the above findings together should make it possible for you to give a definite conclusion about thyroid status although you must be very wary of suggesting either hyper- or hypothyroidism in the presence of a normal pulse. If there remain doubts in your mind after examining the patient, you should be prepared to ask the standard questions about the *symptoms* of thyroid disease (i.e. relating to temperature preference, weight change, appetite, bowel habit, palpitations, and mood changes). This would complete your assessment of the patient's thyroid status.

This patient has diabetes mellitus. Please examine his feet.

Having given you the diagnosis, the examiners will expect you to examine the feet in a logical way, looking in particular for features of the complications of diabetes. After the initial pleasantries, get the patient to lie on the couch and expose his feet and legs. Remember that, at the completion of your examination, you should be able to describe any ulceration or gangrene you observe, and give a good account of any accompanying sensory or vascular changes.

Before concentrating on the feet, look at the patient, from his face downwards, to show the examiner that you do not overlook the general inspection even when you know the diagnosis. Besides, there may be signs present (e.g. cataract, xanthelasmata, dermopathy) that may come up in the discussion.

Skin

Observe any obvious abnormalities such as *ulcers* (neuropathic if found on the sole of the foot over the base of a metatarsal; arterial if found over the lower leg), *missing toes* or any signs of *gangrene* (large vessel disease), or *digital infarcts* (small vessel disease). If you see an ulcer, do not forget to note its dimensions, margins, the presence of slough or discharge on the base, and the state of the surrounding skin. Note the *colour of the skin* (purplish-blue if the circulation is poor), and any *skin lesions* (necrobiosis lipoidica diabeticorum on the anterior shin, granuloma annulare, or any signs of infection). Note whether the feet are of normal *temperature* or are cold, due to poor arterial circulation. There may be loss of hair on the lower legs with shiny skin. Look for any areas of callus over the pressure points.

Look at the ankle joints for any evidence of deformity (*Charcot's joint*), which could indicate sensory loss at the joint from a peripheral neuropathy.

Peripheral pulses

Feel for the dorsalis pedis pulses on both sides and then progress up the legs, feeling the posterior tibial, popliteal and eventually the femoral pulses, comparing right with left each time.

Sensation

The most common sensory defect is a peripheral neuropathy with a 'stocking' distribution. Demonstrate this with light touch (usually the most sensitive indicator) and pinprick. Test first on the trunk to ensure that the patient can appreciate both the touch and the prick. Explain to the patient that you will be testing his leg with the pin from below upwards, and that you would like him to say whether the pinprick remains of the same intensity, becomes duller, or becomes sharper as you go up the leg. Work up the leg to the sensory level where sensation returns or changes and confirm by demonstrating the same level medially and laterally. The level of the peripheral neuropathy may be different on the two legs. Vibration sense should be tested on the medial malleoli. Again, first check that the patient can feel the vibrations from the tuning fork on a bony part assumed to be normal (e.g. the forehead) before asking if he can feel anything over the malleoli.

4.16

Let me introduce you to the lady in this cubicle, Mrs Rafferty (a manikin). She is worried about her breasts and I would like you to examine her.

Even though there is likely to be a manikin at this station, you should treat it as a real person and extend the same courtesy and respect that you would to any female patient. The examination should be conducted with the same thoroughness as you would with a live person. If you are male you should explain to the examiner that you would examine this lady in the presence of a female chaperone.

Introduce yourself to the patient, explain the procedure, and seek her permission to examine her breasts, along the following lines:

> My name is Dr Gupta. I understand that you are worried about your breasts. Please, may I examine you? Would you remove your top clothing so that I can examine your breasts properly? During the procedure you may have to sit up and lie down, but I will try to keep all the moving around or any discomfort to a minimum. Do tell me if any part is particularly tender, so that I will be extra careful. Are you all right? OK.

Examination

Inspection

Sit the patient in a chair and inspect the breasts. For the purposes of a comprehensive examination, divide the breast in your mind into seven parts: the four quadrants, axillary tail, areola, and the nipple (Fig. 4.16.1). Systematically inspect these seven parts and tell the examiner that you are looking for any asymmetry, puckering, or change in the skin colour. Explain that you are

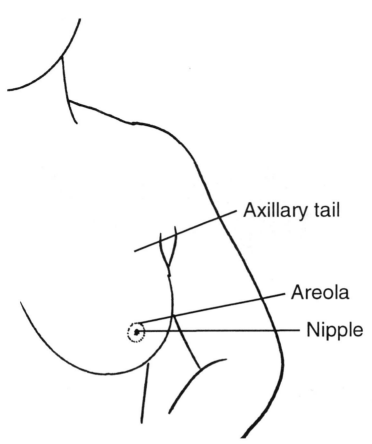

Fig. 4.16.1 Inspection of the breast

looking carefully at the nipple to see if there is a milk scab, suggestive of *galactorrhoea*, or *increased pigmentation of the nipple*, suggestive of Addison's disease (Fig. 4.16.2). Mention that if you found any asymmetry, induration, or swelling, you would get the patient to raise her arms above her head, and then to press her hands firmly on her hips to contract the pectorals. These manoeuvres would make a swelling more visible and show if there was any fixation to the skin or the muscle.

Palpation

Palpate all four quadrants and the axillary tail on each side, with the palm of your hand. Do this with the patient in the resting

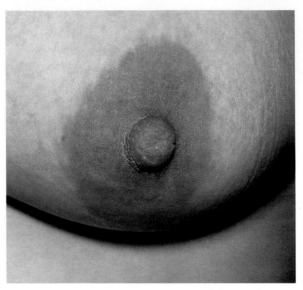

Fig. 4.16.2 Hyperpigmentation of the nipple

position as well as with the patient holding her hands raised above her head (Fig. 4.16.3). As you gently press around the

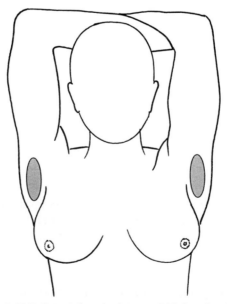

Fig. 4.16.3 Examining the breasts with hands raised

areola, explain to the examiner that you are pressing the glandular tissue against the chest wall to feel for any thickening, nodules, or tenderness.

Next, ask the patient to lie flat on the couch and re-examine all quadrants in each breast. If you feel a swelling you should define its characteristics, such as its size, shape, consistency, tenderness, and whether it is mobile or fixed. Gently hold the areola between your thumb and the index finger and squeeze the palpable ducts to see if there is any galactorrhoea. Lastly, palpate the axillae and pectoral regions for lymph node enlargement. Then thank the patient, and summarize your findings to the examiner.

Please examine this patient's groins.

The patient will need to be unclothed so that the entire inguinal regions and the genitalia are exposed. You should explain the purpose and nature of the examination to the patient and warn him that you may have to stand him up to see if a hernia appears. Although the prime purpose at this station would seem to be to test your technique of examining for a hernia, you should begin by inspecting the lower limbs, groins, and external genitalia for any abrasions, ulcers or swellings. Next, you should palpate the groins.

Examination

Lymph nodes

The inguinal lymph glands are divided into two groups, an oblique set above and beneath and parallel to the inguinal ligament, and a longitudinal set overlying the femoral vessels. These two groups should be palpated on each side. Remember that some of these nodes may be palpable in thin subjects as a normal finding, but they should not be greater than 1 cm in size, tender, or inflamed. If you find any swollen glands note their size, consistency, tenderness, the condition of the overlying skin, and whether they are adherent to the deep structures. Then look again for any primary foci of infection on the legs, groins and genitalia.

Hernias

Hernial protrusion of the abdominal contents occurs at points of weakness. The various types of hernia in this region can be recognized by their position with respect to the pubic tubercle. A *femoral hernia* emerges as a swelling below the inguinal ligament and lateral to the pubic tubercle. An *inguinal hernia* comes

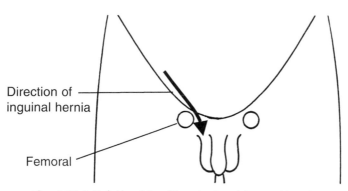

Fig. 4.17.1 Relationship of inguinal and femoral hernias

through the external inguinal ring and lies above and medial to the pubic tubercle (Fig. 4.17.1). An *indirect* inguinal hernia occurs into a persistent remnant of the processus vaginalis. This form of hernia may extend to the testes and often occurs in young men. A *direct* inguinal hernia protrudes through the weakened posterior wall of the inguinal canal lateral to the rectus abdominis muscle. It does not reach the testes and occurs in older men.

If there is a swelling over one of the hernial orifices note its location and grasp it between the thumb and the finger to see if you can get above the swelling. If it is possible to get above it then it is not coming out of the inguinal canal or the abdominal cavity. If it is *not* possible to get above the swelling, note its relationship to, and its continuity with, the inguinal canal. While the neck of the sac is still in your grasp, ask the patient to cough and feel for an impulse.

Reducing a hernia

The next important question to settle is whether a swelling is *reducible*, that is, if it can be returned into the abdominal cavity. Some patients have discovered the art of reducing the hernia themselves and will do so at your request. If the patient complains that the swelling has recently become *irreducible*, then you should *not* attempt to reduce it. If this is not the case, however, and there is no redness over the swelling, you should attempt to reduce it.

Ask the patient to lie on the couch. Flex the hip and the knee to relax the pillars of the superficial inguinal ring. Surround the swelling with the fingers and thumb of one hand like a funnel and *gently* press on the fundus of the swelling with the fingers of the other hand, leading it through the ring. *Do not use excessive force*. While you reduce the swelling you may get an idea of its contents. If the hernia contains omentum it will be easy to reduce and will feel 'doughy'. If it contains the intestine it will be difficult to reduce and you may even hear a gurgle as it returns to the peritoneal cavity.

If there is no obvious swelling you should ask the patient to stand up, turn his head away from you, and give a couple of coughs while you look for a bulge over the hernial orifices. If no bulge appears on coughing then you should keep your fingers on the hernial orifices and ask the patient to cough again — you might then feel an impulse. If there is no swelling and no bulge or impulse on coughing you can conclude that there is no hernia.

Please examine this patient's scrotum.

When you are asked to examine a scrotum, there will usually be a hydrocele. However, you should start with an open mind and fully inspect the (adequately exposed) external genitalia in good light, before you palpate all the contents of the scrotum (testes, tunica vaginalis, epididymis, spermatic cord, and the superficial inguinal ring). As usual, you should introduce yourself to the patient and seek his permission for the examination.

Stand the patient in good light while you sit facing him. If there is no swelling the contour of the testes will be visible, with the left testis hanging fractionally lower. If the scrotal sac looks swollen ascertain whether there is soft, pitting oedema (e.g. in congestive cardiac failure or nephrotic syndrome) or fluid in the tunica vaginalis (a hydrocele). Look for any signs of cellulitis, or tethering of the scrotum due to testicular disease (tumour, tuberculosis).

Gently palpate the body of the testes and compare them. The tunica vaginalis is blended anteriorly with the testes. Palpate the epididymis, its body, globus major (head) and globus minor (tail). To feel the spermatic cord, pass the index finger under the neck of the scrotum, and pinch the underlying structures between the thumb and the finger. You will be able to slip the constituents of the scrotum through your fingers from within outwards. You ought to be able to find the vas which feels like hard whipcord. You will also feel nerves and the fibres of the cremaster muscle. Look out for any thickening or tenderness.

Next, determine the *translucency* of the scrotal sac. If there is an intrascrotal swelling, make it tense by grasping the neck of the scrotum between the fingers and thumb. Apply a lit pocket torch to the distal side of the swelling. In most cystic swellings the entire sac will light up. In a large, tense hydrocele the testis may not have been easily palpable, but will become apparent on transillumination as a dark oval shadow posteriorly. Transillumination is the essential feature for a diagnosis of hydocele.

Have a look at this swelling and then examine it to arrive at a diagnosis.

The examination of a lump is one of the most elementary skills and you will need to give a good account of yourself by following all the steps in the correct sequence. Before you touch the swelling, ask the patient if it is painful or tender. Be gentle throughout and reassure the patient that you will be careful not to hurt him.

Location

Inspect the swelling, note its location, and look for any signs of inflammation over and around it. A lipoma may arise anywhere on the body and they are often multiple. A cavernous haemangioma arises in the orbit and is compressible (see below). A malignant melanoma can arise in any pigmented tissue, usually in a pigmented mole — in males the commonest site is the trunk, and in females, the legs.

Anatomical plane

Determine the exact anatomical plane in which the swelling is situated. It may be in the skin (sebaceous cyst, abscess); subcutaneous (lipoma, neuroma, neurofibroma); in the muscle; over a tendon (ganglion); arising from a bone (tumour); or attached to an organ. A cutaneous swelling will move with the skin; subcutaneous swellings will move a little in every direction without moving the skin. A swelling in a muscle can be moved when the muscle is relaxed and is fixed when the muscle is contracted. A bony tumour, such as a sarcoma or a secondary tumour, cannot be moved away from the site of its origin.

Physical characteristics

Examine the swelling carefully and gently in order to discern the various physical characteristics of the lump. Avoid palpating deeply if it is very tender.

1. *Size.* Measure the dimensions of the swelling using a tape measure.
2. *Shape.* Is it spherical or flattened; regular, or irregular and knobbly?
3. *Margin.* Does it have a well-defined margin or does it merge with the surrounding tissues? If it is irregular, feel whether it is lobulated (e.g. a lipoma lying superficial to the deep fascia) by steadying the swelling with one hand and feeling the structure with the index finger of the other hand. As you press firmly with your finger the swelling may slip under the finger, the so-called 'slipping' sign that is a characteristic feature of a subcutaneous lipoma.
4. *Consistency.* Determine whether the swelling is *cystic* (containing fluid) or *solid* by gently dipping the tip of your index finger on the surface to see if there is any 'give' as the fluid under the finger is displaced. In cystic swellings you can elicit two further signs, *fluctuation* and *transillumination.* To demonstrate fluctuation steady the swelling between your middle finger and thumb and tap the surface at one end, noting whether the impulse is transmitted to a finger placed at the opposite end. A tense, cystic swelling may not exhibit fluctuation, however, and the procedure should not even be attempted if the swelling is acutely tender. You can elicit transillumination by placing the lit end of a pen torch at one end of the swelling — it will light up if the fluid is either clear or haemorrhagic.

    If the swelling is not cystic determine whether it is soft, firm like a contracted muscle, or bony hard. Attempt to indent the surface of the swelling. If the depression remains, the swelling may contain viscid material (e.g. a large dermoid or sebaceous cyst, impacted faeces in the sigmoid colon).
5. *Compressibility.* If the swelling is a cavernous haemangioma or a lymphangioma it can be compressed and emptied, either fully or partially, and it will refill gradually. A cystic swelling with a narrow neck, such as a meningocele, would also exhibit this sign.

339

6. *Pulsation.* If the swelling is pulsatile it is important to determine whether it is transmitting the pulsations of a neighbouring artery or is itself pulsating. Place your index fingers on either side of the swelling and see if the fingers move parallel to each other with each pulsation (a transmitted pulse) or away from each other (a pulsatile swelling, e.g. aneurysm, arteriovenous fistula).

7. *Sounds.* You may be able to hear a systolic bruit over an aneurysm or a continuous murmur (i.e. through systole and diastole) over an arteriovenous fistula.

Some swellings are diagnosable from their appearance and physical characteristics (e.g. melanoma, cavernous haemangioma, lipoma, sebaceous and dermoid cysts, neurofibroma). However, in these and in all other cases, you should be able to give a complete description of the swelling, stating where the swelling is originating from; whether it is mobile or fixed to the skin or the underlying structures; whether it is smooth, irregular, or lobulated; whether it is soft, firm, or hard; and whether it is transmitting pulsations or is intrinsically pulsatile. With a little more thought, you should be able to add whether it is congenital or acquired, inflammatory, traumatic, or neoplastic.

Please examine this ulcer and summarize your findings.

The examiner has asked you to give him your findings and you should present these in the orthodox sequence of: site, size, shape, edge, floor, base, discharge, surrounding tissues, and the draining lymph nodes. Keeping to this sequence will also help you to develop some diagnostic hypotheses as you go along. Once you have introduced yourself to the patient, ask him if the ulcer or the area surrounding it is painful. Reassure him that you will try not to hurt him.

Examination

General

Look at the patient to get some idea of his general state of health and nutrition. He may look thin and wasted (neoplasia, chronic infection, inflammatory bowel disease) or may show discoloration of the face, hands, or feet (peripheral vascular disease). If he is obese he might have type II diabetes mellitus and an ulcer on the foot might be related to the underlying condition. This survey should not take longer than a few seconds and you should quickly move on to examine the ulcer itself.

The ulcer

1. *Site.* The location of an ulcer is often an important clue to the diagnosis. A rodent ulcer (basal cell carcinoma of the skin) commonly occurs on the middle one-third of the face, usually on the nose or forehead. Varicose and stasis ulcers are often found on the legs (Fig. 4.20.1 and Fig. 4.20.2). Arterial ulcers may also be found on the legs, usually above the lateral malleolus or on the shin (Fig. 4.20.3). An arterial ulcer is

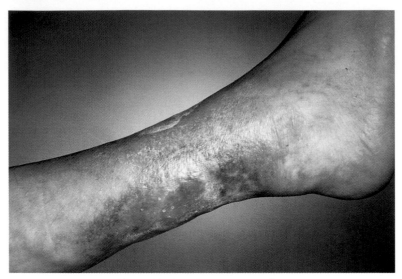

Fig. 4.20.1 Varicose venous ulcer

often painful and associated with absent pedal pulses. A neuropathic ulcer (also known as a *trophic*, perforating or pressure ulcer) characteristically occurs on the plantar surface of the foot at the base of the big toe.

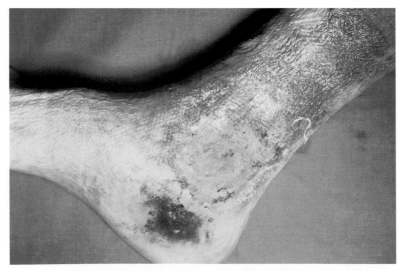

Fig. 4.20.2 Stasis ulcer

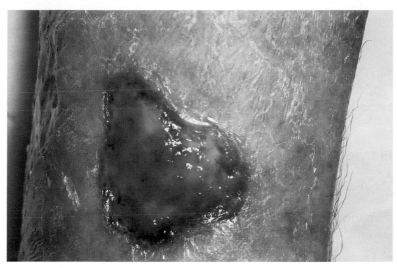

Fig. 4.20.3 Well-defined margin and slough-covered base

2. *Size*. Use a tape measure to determine the transverse and vertical dimensions of the ulcer.
3. *Shape*. The ulcer may be round, oval, irregular or serpiginous (advancing, leaving behind a healing area).
4. *Edge*. The appearance of the edge gives you important information about the nature of the ulcer. The edges may be *everted* and hard, as in a carcinomatous ulcer; *raised*, as in a rodent ulcer; *undermined*, as in a tuberculous ulcer; or *sloping*, as in a varicose ulcer. Trophic ulcers have *punched-out* edges and pyoderma gangrenosum has oedematous and undermined edges.
5. *Base*. Examine the base to see if there is any slough (Fig. 4.20.3), scab, exudate, or pus. In some arterial ulcers the underlying structures, such as tendons and muscles, are exposed. Gently feel the base to see if it is indurated or attached to the deeper structures. (Wash your hands afterwards.)
6. *Surrounding tissues*. Look for signs of inflammation, oedema, pigmentation, and, in the lower limbs, varicose veins.
7. *Regional lymph glands*. Complete the examination by feeling the regional lymph nodes. If glands are enlarged note their size, any tenderness, and signs of inflammation.

Please examine this patient's nose.

This is a fairly straightforward task but its simplicity and rarity seem to unsettle candidates in the examination. Some candidates even miss one of the three main components of the examination routine:

- External inspection
- Nasal cavities
- Nasopharynx

External inspection

Even if the subject is a manikin you must not miss this step — the nose may provide useful clues to a systemic disorder. A large, fleshy nose may be seen in normal subjects but, together with other relevant facial features, is characteristically seen in acromegaly. Nasal tumours, polyps or granulomata (Wegener's granulomatosis) may alter the shape of the nose and may be easily seen on inspection of the nasal cavities. In Wegener's granulomatosis there is sometimes a reddish hue on the nose overlying the granulomata.

A depressed nasal bridge is a cardinal sign of congenital syphilis though this condition is rarely seen these days. A purple-red infiltration of part of the nose (*lupus pernio*) is seen in sarcoidosis. Lupus vulgaris is a rare form of cutaneous tuberculosis and may involve the nose with brownish-red nodules which may ulcerate and cause scarring. Other cutaneous disorders, such as pemphigus, erysipelas, and systemic lupus erythematosus may also involve the nose and the face.

Nasal cavities

Lift the tip of the nose gently with your left thumb and inspect the anterior passages. In an adult you will need a speculum to

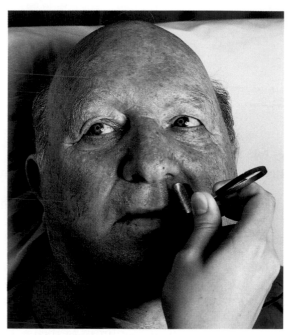

Fig. 4.21.1 Introducing a nasal speculum

view the interior of each nasal cavity. Introduce the closed speculum gently (Fig. 4.21.1) and allow the prongs to separate to get a good view. There may be a tumour, granulomata, mucosal swelling (vasomotor or allergic rhinitis), or displacement or dislocation of the septum. See if there is any discharge and whether it is clear and watery or mucopurulent.

Nasopharynx

The posterior nasal cavities and the upper pharynx can be viewed with a postnasal mirror. Warm the mirror to prevent any condensation forming and advance it beyond the soft palate to view the posterior nasal passages. This procedure may reveal hypertrophied turbinates (allergic rhinitis), adenoids, or the presence of a nasopharyngeal carcinoma.

Examine Mr Hopkirk's right knee. He has sustained an injury to it while playing rugby.

Although it is clear that your knee joint examination skills are being tested here and that you will have to carry out a comprehensive examination, you should be on the lookout for the various specific signs of a deranged knee. For example, the examiners will be watching to see if you can test the stability of the knee joint, irrespective of the presence of any obvious signs of an injury. You should also remember that having sustained an injury in no way disqualifies Mr Hopkirk from having some pre-existing knee disease, such as osteoarthrosis or rheumatoid arthritis. Before you start you should briefly review in your own mind the possible conditions that might be present:

- Damage resulting from injury
  — Meniscus lesions
  — Rupture of anterior or posterior cruciate ligaments
  — Loose bodies
  — Osteochondral fracture
  — Effusion
- Swelling of the knee joint
  — Osteoarthrosis
  — Rheumatoid arthritis
  — Ankylosing spondylitis
  — Psoriatic arthritis
  — Gout or pseudogout
  — Haemarthrosis

Examination

Inspection and palpation are the two chief components of the examination of the knee joint. Inspection is a very important part of this examination and it is best conducted while the patient is wearing shorts or briefs, which allows you to have a good view of the knee joints as well as the thigh muscles.

Inspection

Ask the patient to stand with his knees together while you inspect them both from the front and the back. The knee should be in straight line with the hip and ankle joints. Look for any lateral angulation (genu valgum, Fig. 4.22.1) or medial angulation (genu varum); any swelling (Fig. 4.22.2) and its extent; and for the presence of normal landmarks such as the patella and parapatellar grooves. These will be obscured and there may even be a bulge if there is an effusion. Look for any scars or redness of the skin. Cystic swelling of the menisci, if present, will be seen in the anteromedial and lateral regions of the joint. There may be a swelling anteriorly due to prepatellar

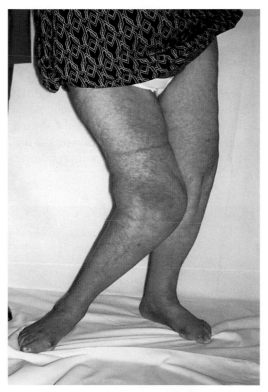

Fig. 4.22.1 Genu valgum

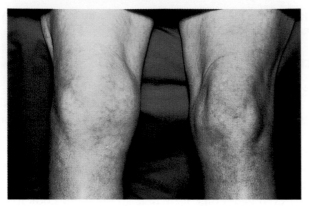

Fig. 4.22.2 Effusion of the right knee

bursitis (housemaid's knee), or posteriorly due to rupture of a popliteal cyst (Baker's cyst).

Palpation

Palpation is best done with the patient lying supine, the knee extended and the quadriceps femoris adequately relaxed. With your left hand placed about 10 cm above the patella, push gently downwards to feel the consistency, thickness, nodularity, or swelling of the suprapatellar pouch, which may be palpable due to synovitis, effusion, or a tumour. Palpate the synovial membrane by grasping the patella and pressing it onto the femoral condyles to see if there is any pain, tenderness, crepitus, or grating (Fig. 4.22.3).

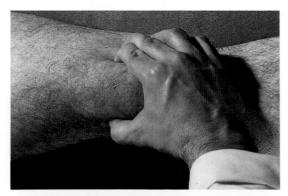

Fig. 4.22.3 Feeling the synovial membrane

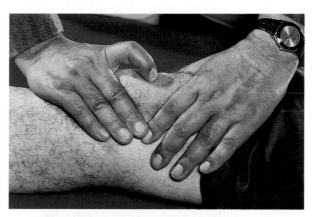

Fig. 4.22.4 Demonstrating the patellar tap

A large synovial effusion is easy to recognize as it forms a characteristic horseshoe-shaped swelling around the patella. Using both hands you should be able to elicit cross fluctuation and demonstrate the presence of fluid by tapping the patella (Fig. 4.22.4). Small effusions are detected by the *bulge sign.* You can perform this test by forcing fluid out of the suprapatellar pouch with your left hand, while steadying the patella with your index finger. As you stroke down the groove between the patella and the femoral condyles with your right hand, you will see a bulge in the opposite groove caused by the displaced fluid.

Tenderness localized to either the medial or the lateral aspect of the tibiofemoral joint line suggests a tear or damage of the meniscus or the corresponding collateral ligament. An injury to the meniscus or active arthritis will limit extension and the patient will tend to walk on his toes with the knee flexed at about 15° (Fig. 4.22.5). You may have noticed this as the patient was walking.

Stability
The precise cause of internal derangement can be diagnosed and the stability of the knee joint can be tested using the following manoeuvres:

1. *Abduction test.* Stabilize the femur with one hand to prevent its abduction while you abduct the tibia with the other hand (Fig. 4.22.6). This manoeuvre will compress the lateral meniscus and cause pain if it is damaged. The same procedure

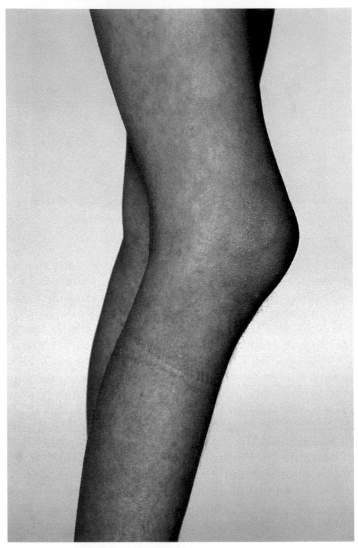

Fig. 4.22.5 Pain limiting full extension of the knee

will also stretch the medial collateral ligament and cause pain if that is damaged.

2. *Adduction test.* Once again, stabilize the femur with one hand and adduct the tibia with the other hand. This test will reveal injuries of the medial meniscus and the lateral collateral ligament.

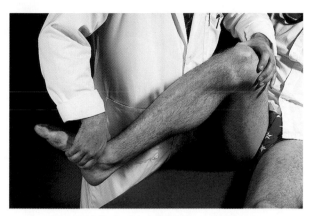

Fig. 4.22.6 Testing abduction of the knee

3. *McMurray test*. This is a combination of the above two tests and is frequently used for detecting internal derangement of the knee. Place one hand over the anterior aspect of the fully flexed knee with the index finger placed along the line of the tibiofemoral joint on one side and the thumb on the other. Now grasp the ankle with the other hand and flex the knee while you rotate the leg laterally (Fig. 4.22.7) and medially.

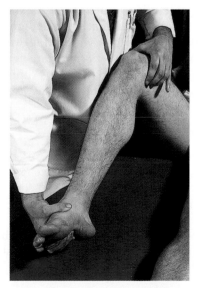

Fig. 4.22.7 The McMurray test

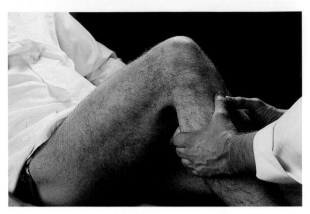

Fig. 4.22.8 Testing the anterior cruciate ligament

You may hear a click or a pop, from a torn meniscus, during full flexion and internal or external rotation. The patellofemoral abnormalities will cause grating or crepitation during extension.

4. *Anterior drawer or Lachman test.* This and the next manoeuvre will test the anteroposterior stability of the knee (cruciate ligaments). Semi-flex the knee and pull the tibia forwards (Fig. 4.22.8). The anterior cruciate ligament holds the tibia back. If this ligament is ruptured then the tibia will be lying anterior to the straight line that should align it with the patella, and it will yield when you pull forwards.

5. *Posterior drawer test.* The posterior cruciate ligament holds the tibia forwards in line with the femur. Its rupture will cause the tibia to sag backwards and it will 'give' as you press it back (Fig. 4.22.9).

Movements
Flexion of the knee is limited to 135° to 150° by the muscular bulk of the thigh and calf. The normal knee extends to a straight line and it can be hyperextended up to 15°. Test both passive and active movements while you are performing the stability tests.

Feel the popliteal space, in the standing and the prone positions, for tenderness, bursitis, a popliteal cyst, and spasm of the hamstring muscles.

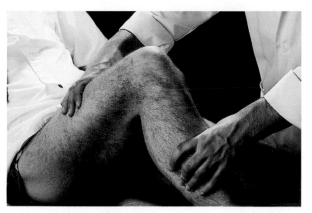

Fig. 4.22.9 Testing the posterior cruciate ligament

Muscular bulk

During your inspection you would have looked to see if there was any evidence of atrophy of the quadriceps and hamstring muscles. Now make an objective assessment of any atrophy. With both knees fully extended, mark a spot about 20 cm above the tibial tubercle on both thighs, and measure their girth with a tape measure. Muscle atrophy is confirmed if the bulk is reduced by more than 1 cm on the affected side.

This patient is complaining of pain in his right hip. Please examine his hip joints.

The pain may originate in the hip or may be referred from the lower spine from a prolapsed intervertebral disc. Even if the patient is a normal volunteer you should be able to discuss the following conditions which may cause pain in the hip:

- Osteoarthrosis
- Rheumatoid arthritis
- Ankylosing spondylitis
- Reiter's syndrome
- Pyogenic arthritis
- Primary bone tumour
- Irritable hip — transient synovitis

You must also bear in mind special conditions which affect the hip in children and in the elderly.

Children

- *Congenital dislocation of the hip.* Characterized by disturbance of gait and posture and shortening of the corresponding limb. It may present in adults if it has not been treated adequately in early childhood.
- *Slipped femoral epiphysis.* The femoral head slips down, causing external rotation, adduction, and shortening of the limb. It is common in boys.
- *Perthes' disease.* Osteonecrosis or osteochondrosis of the femoral head.

The elderly

- *Fractured neck of the femur.* This is usually an acute event caused by trauma and presents with pain and difficulty in weight bearing.

■ *Complications of hip replacement.* Component fracture, usually in obese subjects, infection and component loosening.

Although you will be expected to know the main features of these conditions, it is unlikely that candidates will see many of these in the PLAB exam. It is equally unlikely that you will be required to carry out a detailed orthopaedic assessment, but you should be familiar with and be able to demonstrate the principal components of such an examination.

Examination

Inspection, both in standing and lying positions, observation of gait and movements, and the assessment of muscular bulk and power are the chief components of the examination of the hip. The patient should be wearing only briefs so that you have an adequate view of the bony prominences and musculature.

Inspection

1. Get the patient to stand facing you, with his legs together, and look for any *pelvic tilting.* During the inspection routine you should be able to get a good idea of whether any pelvic tilting present is caused by scoliosis, a short leg, adduction/abduction deformity of the hip, muscular wasting (secondary to infection, disuse, or polio), or osteoarthrosis.
2. Ask the patient to turn to his side so that you can have a side view of his hip and spine. This is an ideal way to reveal exaggerated *lordosis,* which is suggestive of a fixed-flexion deformity of the hip.
3. Next, get the patient to turn his back to you to allow you to look at his back for any *scoliosis,* which may be a primary (congenital) cause of pelvic tilt. Look for any *gluteal wasting* (infection, disuse) and for any sinus scars from old tuberculosis.
4. *Gait* — watch the patient walk from the front, side and behind. Note if the strides are full, rhythmic and regular, and if there is any pain, limp, or tilting.
5. Ask the patient to lie supine on the couch with his legs straight and the feet held together. Look at the level of the iliac spines (a transverse line running across the superior iliac spines) and the heel level. If there is no *shortening* (apparent or

real) of either leg the heels will be at the same level and the line joining the iliac spines will be at a right angle to the edge of the couch. If there is any pelvic tilting suggestive of shortening of a limb, then you will need to determine whether it is apparent or real, and whether the shortening is below or above the greater trochanter.

Palpation

Shortening

The *true leg length* is the distance between the anterior iliac spine and the inferior border of the corresponding medial malleolus. The *apparent leg length* is the distance between the umbilicus and the same point on the medial malleolus. Any *apparent shortening* may be due to adduction contracture compensated by pelvic tilting.

True shortening of the leg can be determined by comparing the length on the side of the pelvic tilt to the length of the opposite leg. If one leg *is* shorter you should determine if it is due to shortening above the trochanter (fractured neck of femur, infection, Perthes' disease): hook your thumbs just below the anterior iliac spines on both sides and palpate the greater trochanters posteriorly with your fingers, estimating the distance between the forefinger and the thumb on both sides. The distance will be narrower on the side of shortening above the trochanter.

Measure the length of the femur from the greater trochanter to the line of the knee joint and compare it with the opposite leg. Next, measure the length of the tibia from the line of the knee joint to the inferior border of the medial malleolus and compare it with the opposite leg.

These measurements will allow you to decide whether there is true or apparent shortening, and, if there is true shortening, whether it is due to a cause above the trochanter or due to a shorter femur or a shorter tibia.

Tenderness and swelling

Ask the patient to point out any areas of pain and feel these for tenderness, soft-tissue swelling, and for evidence of inflammation. Apply firm pressure behind and superiorly over the greater trochanter, which may be tender if the neighbouring synovial membrane is inflamed or contains fluid.

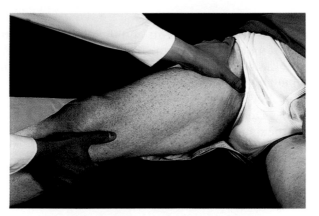

Fig. 4.23.1 Palpating the lesser trochanter

To feel the lesser trochanter, rotate the leg externally and palpate just below the medial third of the inguinal ligament (Fig. 4.23.1). The lesser trochanter may be tender from strains of the iliopsoas muscle resulting from athletic injuries. Semi-flex the knee and abduct the thigh and then ask the patient to bring the leg closer to the midline as you feel for the origin of adductor longus below the midpoint of the inguinal ligament (Fig. 4.23.2). This is sometimes inflamed in sports personnel, and you would also be able to feel the adductor contracture that occurs in osteoarthrosis of the hip joint. Feel posteriorly over the ischial tuberosity, which is usually tender in ischiogluteal bursitis (*weaver's bottom*), and note any swelling in this area.

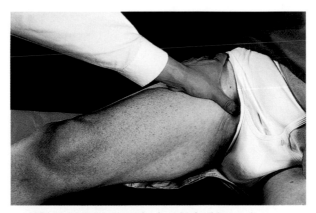

Fig. 4.23.2 Feeling the head of adductor longus

Movements

Test passive and active movements and thereby the integrity of the muscles responsible for them. The pelvic contribution to movements can be neutralized by steadying the iliac crest firmly while you test passive movement with the other hand. Extension of the thigh should be tested while the patient lies on the opposite side. During abduction, pelvic movement is checked by a hand on the opposite iliac crest. Look for any signs of pain or limitation of movement during these manoeuvres.

Little Laura's mother has brought her in to Casualty because she is not feeling well. Please examine her.

You are not given the age of the child but if it is a manikin the examiner may tell you this as he introduces you to the patient and her mother. Remember, even if it is a manikin, you will be expected to observe all the usual niceties and courtesies.

Examining a child

Do not separate an infant from her mother and do not undress her. Involve the mother in the process and she will be able to expose the relevant part for you. You can often examine a sleeping infant without causing her too much inconvenience.

If it is an older child engage her in conversation, ask her about her interests, hobbies, or favourite toys, and then explain every step of the examination, asking for her permission. Often, it is easier and more diplomatic to give the child a choice in the proceedings, for example, 'I have to examine your chest and heart. Which one would you like me to examine first?'

Your hands and the implements you touch the child with must be warm. Leave the uncomfortable procedures (e.g. otoscopy, examination of the oropharynx and fundi) to the last (even if the patient is a manikin). Show care and consideration for the child's dignity. Cover the parts that have been examined or are yet to be examined. Offer words of encouragement in between various steps (That's brilliant!, You are doing fine!, Well done! etc.) and thank her after completing each procedure.

Inspection

This is the most important part of the paediatric examination. You should have a set plan in your head although you do not need to follow it in the same sequence each time.

1. *General.* Look at the general state of the child, whether she looks ill, uncomfortable, or in pain, and whether her appearance, height, and weight are in keeping with her age and sex. Form an impression of the child's state of nutrition and hydration (marasmus); the colour and texture of her skin (pallor, icterus, cyanosis, rashes); and whether there are any abnormalities in her posture (hypotonia, muscular dystrophy, musculoskeletal deformity) or gait (waddling, spastic, hypotonic).

2. *Head.* In a young infant you should look at the size and shape, for moulding and the presence of a cephalhaematoma or bossing, and at the state of the fontanelles, skin, veins, and hair. In all children you have to consider if the size of the skull is inappropriately large (hydrocephalus) and if there is any asymmetry or area of unusual prominence.

3. *Face.* Look for any asymmetry and to see whether the mandibles and maxillary bones are underdeveloped. Look at the eyes. There may be photophobia, nystagmus, exophthalmos, discharge, and abnormally set eyes or palpebral fissures. Check the size and shape of the pupils, the colour of the iris and sclera, and whether there are corneal opacities. Note any purulent nasal discharge.

4. *Oropharynx.* Note the colour of the lips and look for the presence of any fissures, the state of oral hygiene, and whether the adenoids or tonsils are congested or enlarged.

5. *Ears.* Note the position and shape of the ears and look to see if there is any discharge.

6. *Neck.* Look for any deviation (torticollis) and for the presence of webbing or any swelling.

7. *Trunk.* Note the shape and symmetry of the ribcage; the spinal curvature and the position of the scapulae; the position and state of the nipples and umbilicus; any pulsations over the precordium and epigastrium; indrawing of the supraclavicular fossae and intercostal spaces; any visible peristalsis over the abdomen; and any swellings over the chest, abdomen, or at the hernial orifices. Look at the condition of the external genitalia.

8. *Extremities*. Look for any deformities, swellings, extra digits, the state of the nails, and for any abnormal movements (chorea or choreoathetosis).

Palpation, percussion and auscultation

Record the height, weight, and head circumference. Feel the neck, axillae, and the inguinal regions for lymph nodes, and any other swelling you may have noted on inspection. In infants it is convenient and expeditious for the child and the mother to combine the examination of the respiratory and cardiovascular systems and the abdomen by examining first the front and then the back — palpate, percuss, and auscultate the chest and abdomen at the front and then repeat these procedures over the back.

The nervous system

You may have already noticed any wasting, asymmetry, abnormal movements, or abnormality of gait. Now check the tone and power in the upper and lower extremities and test the tendon and superficial reflexes. This basic screening neurological examination may be all that is required but bear in mind that if there is any abnormality then you would have to go on to perform a more in-depth examination to explore it.

This is Mrs Summers (a manikin) who is 37 years old. She is 8 weeks pregnant and I would like you to proceed with a booking visit assessment.

It is clear from the instructions that this is the initial booking examination. As the midwife carries out most of the initial antenatal examination, you will have to wait to see what particular skills the examiner wants to test you on. At this stage you should proceed to explain and perform a comprehensive clinical assessment. You should start by telling the examiner how you would examine the patient, explaining each aspect briefly.

History and pregnancy planning

You would:

- Establish the accuracy of the gestation duration by comparing the date of the last menstrual period with an ultrasound scan
- Discuss any past and present medical problems
- Discuss screening tests for Down's syndrome and other conditions
- Plan pregnancy visits, shared care, and midwifery-led care

Examination

- Height and weight
- Blood pressure
- Oral hygiene and mucous membranes
- Heart and lungs
- Abdominal palpation
- Urinalysis (for proteinuria and glycosuria)

The midwife will have recorded the height and weight, as in any routine medical examination. The blood pressure should be recorded after a few minutes' rest, with the patient supine. The diastolic blood pressure should be taken both at phase 4 (when the Korotkoff sounds muffle) and at phase 5, when the sounds disappear (see p. 385). In some pregnant patients, as the pregnancy advances, the sounds may not disappear and you may have to rely on the phase 4 recordings.

The face and mucosal surfaces should be looked at for any evidence of discoloration (pallor, icterus, or cyanosis). The mouth should be examined to assess the general state of dentition and oral hygiene. Pregnancy is often associated with *hypertrophic gingivitis* and women should be given appropriate advice about dental hygiene before the hypertrophy starts. A mild degree of *thyroid enlargement* is normal in pregnancy, but heat intolerance and resting tachycardia should arouse a suspicion of hyperthyroidism.

A careful examination of the heart may be necessary if there is any history of a cardiac problem. *Flow murmurs* due to increased blood volume and flow are common in pregnancy and are not of any clinical significance.

The abdomen should be palpated to detect the presence of any organ enlargement. The uterus becomes palpable suprapubically at 12 weeks' gestation.

Ask for a urine specimen to test for protein and sugar.

This is Mrs Randall (a manikin). She is 34 weeks pregnant and has come for a follow-up visit. I would like you to examine her for a general assessment.

It is clear that the pregnancy is in an advanced stage, but the examiner is not asking you to perform a specific obstetric examination here (see p. 442). You are being tested on your overall clinical assessment of a pregnant lady attending for a routine follow-up visit. You should start by introducing yourself to Mrs Randall and then explain to the examiner and to the patient what you are going to do.

In a general assessment in an obstetric case you should:

- Ask about her general state of health and any problems that have arisen recently
- Enquire about fetal movements
- Ask if she has any queries
- Measure the blood pressure
- Examine the heart and lungs (if there is a pre-existing lesion or if indicated by the history)
- Palpate the abdomen
- Examine the legs
- Perform urinalysis

While you explain the various steps of the examination to the examiner and the patient, have a look at the patient with regard to her general state of health and nutrition. Look at the mucous membranes for pallor or any other discoloration. Many women, particularly of darker complexions, develop pigmentation over the forehead and cheeks (chloasma).

By now the patient will have rested for a couple of minutes and you can measure her blood pressure (see p. 385). As mentioned in the last case the diastolic blood pressure should be taken both at phase 4 and phase 5. In late pregnancy the blood pressure should be recorded in the lateral supine position to avoid compression of the inferior vena cava. In some patients, adopting the direct supine position may cause hypotension and even syncope and nausea, a condition known as the *supine hypotensive syndrome.*

The abdominal wall commonly shows stretch marks (striae gravidarum). The linea alba, which extends from the umbilicus to the symphysis pubis, becomes pigmented (linea nigra). Examine the legs, looking for oedema and varicose veins.

Although a detailed obstetric examination is not required, you should palpate the abdomen. Locate the fundus of the uterus and measure the distance from the fundus to the symphysis pubis with a tape measure. The uterus becomes palpable suprapubically at 12 weeks' gestation; by 20 weeks it reaches the level of the umbilicus; and at 36 weeks the uterine fundus reaches the level of the xiphisternum and remains at this height until term. You may also be able to determine the lie of the fetus (see p. 442). Complete the examination by palpating for the other intra-abdominal organs.

Thank the patient and help her to get up from the couch.

You are an SHO in Casualty where Mr Phillips presents with pain in his back after having fallen at a building site. Please examine and advise him.

At this station, there will be an actor who will tell you that he has fallen off a building and is now having severe pain in his back. You will be expected to take a brief history from him; examine him (explaining each step to the examiner); arrange an X-ray of his back; reassure him that there is no bony injury; arrange physiotherapy for him; and prescribe a painkiller to relieve his pain.

Take a brief history, asking him to describe what happened, and get him to show you any areas of pain or tenderness.

Examination

In your examination you should check the following:

- *Head and neck.* Look for any bruises, swellings, fractures, and bleeding.
- *Otoscopy.* Look in the ear canals for any bleeding.
- *Nasal cavities.* Check for any bleeding or evidence of a fracture.
- *Oropharynx.* Look for any blood or broken teeth.
- *Neck movements.* See whether he can move his neck freely or if there is any restriction or pain on movement.
- *Arms.* Ask him to move them to reveal any disability, pain, or restriction of movement. Look for bruises and swellings.
- *Chest.* Look, and then palpate, for any swelling or tenderness suggestive of a rib fracture.
- *Groins and legs.* Look for swelling and bruises. Check leg movements.
- *Back.* Look for swellings and bruises, and palpate the spinal processes for any tenderness. Check flexion, extension, and

lateral bending and look for any signs of pain or restriction of movement.

Arrange an X-ray of the spine and once the film is back, have a chat with the patient:

Doctor: Mr Phillips, thank you for your cooperation. I am pleased to say that the X-rays show that there is no bony injury.

Mr Phillips: But I am dying from the pain! Can't you give me something for it?

Doctor: When you fell on your back you injured some of the soft tissues and that is the cause of your pain. I will give you a painkiller which should relieve it, but if the pain does persist please come back to see me.

Mr Phillips: Thank you, doctor.

Practical procedures

Introduction

Success in the PLAB exam makes a doctor eligible to practise safely as a Senior House Officer in a first appointment in a UK hospital. The content of this exam reflects the standard laid down by the General Medical Council for granting limited registration. Registered doctors must be proficient in certain procedures they would be expected to perform as Senior House Officers in the UK. You will be asked to perform at least three procedures in this exam.

In this section we have presented 26 practical procedures that we expect a Senior House Officer to be able to perform, though some of them, such as inserting a chest drain would require supervision. You will be expected to be quite proficient in some of the minor procedures, such as intravenous injections, venous cannulation, arterial puncture, and the correct completion of request forms and labelling of bottles. You may already have acquired some of these skills but we suggest that you should study them carefully and practise them on a manikin repeatedly until you are able to do them skilfully and efficiently.

The purpose of practising the procedures (even those you think you already know) is to make you less liable to clumsiness caused by exam nerves. When the procedure is completed remember always to clean up carefully, collect any rubbish and put it in the bin, and put all sharp objects in the sharps bin. The examiner is watching not only how you perform a procedure, but also how methodical, careful, and *safe* you are.

This patient has just collapsed. Perform cardiopulmonary resuscitation (CPR) on him.

The purpose of this station is to test your resuscitation skills and the instruction may be phrased in a variety of ways: you may be asked to revive or resuscitate a collapsed patient for example. This is a *compulsory* station and every candidate will have to pass it. Failure to satisfy the examiner in this task will cost you a place on the pass list. You should master the sequence of steps given here and be able to go through them without hesitation or confusion about what to do next. The examiner may ask you to explain each of your steps but he will not interfere.

1. As soon as you hear the instruction rush to the collapsed patient who will be a manikin. Before you go too close, make sure that it is safe for you and for the patient. Ask the examiner if it is safe to approach. Appear calm, do not dither, gently shake the manikin, and shout, 'Hello, are you all right?' (Fig. 5.1.1).
2. There will be no response. Shout for help if you are supposed to be in a street (so that some passer-by hears you). In the exam setting, ask the examiner to ring for an ambulance (or for the CPR team if the examiner has indicated that you are on a ward).
3. Perform the standard *ABC* check: *A* for airway, *B* for breathing and *C* for circulation. Check the *airway* by extending the neck and pulling the jaw forward (Fig. 5.1.2). Look in the mouth and oropharynx for any visible obstruction, and leave well-fitting dentures in place. Remove all vomitus and loose teeth.
4. Check the *breathing* for 10 seconds by looking at the chest wall for any rise with inspiration. Simultaneously, feel for any breath on your cheek and listen carefully for any breath sounds. If there is no breathing, and you are in a street,

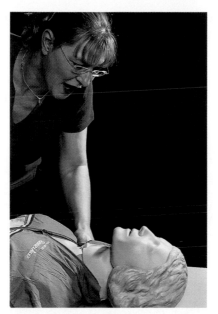

Fig. 5.1.1 Trying to elicit a response in a collapsed patient

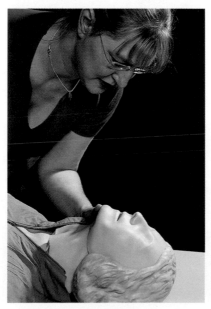

Fig. 5.1.2 Checking the airway

make sure help is arriving — otherwise you may have to go and get help.

With the airway kept open, block the nose with your left thumb and index finger, and give two effective mouth-to-mouth breaths (Fig. 5.1.3). Ensure a good seal around the lips. If the two breaths are ineffective give up to five.

5. Now check the *circulation* by feeling the carotid pulse for 10 seconds (Fig. 5.1.4).

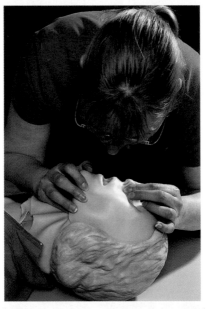

Fig. 5.1.3 Preparing for mouth-to-mouth

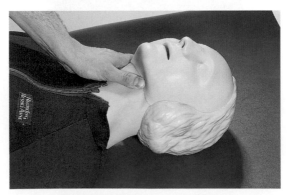

Fig. 5.1.4 Feeling the carotid pulse

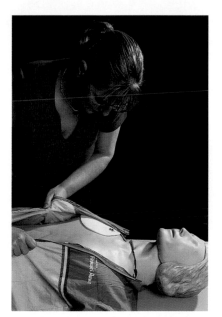

Fig. 5.1.5 Exposing the chest

6. If there is no pulse or breathing (explain this to the examiner), tear off the shirt to expose the chest (Fig. 5.1.5). If there is no pulse, start CPR. If the collapse was witnessed you can then deliver a blow to the precordium. With the hands over the lower part of the sternum (Fig. 5.1.6), start compressing the sternum to a depth of *5 to 6 cm* at a rate of 100 per minute. The ratio of chest compressions to ventilation is the same whether there are one or two 'rescuers', that is, 15 compressions to 2 breaths. Continue CPR until *advanced life support* becomes available, which will include a defibrillator, a drug tray, and oxygen.

7. Connect the monitor leads to the manikin and assess the rhythm, which may be ventricular fibrillation/tachycardia, in which case you can proceed to deliver a shock to cardiovert; or it may be asystole, when no shock will be necessary. (Observe, then explain if the examiner had asked you to, and then act.)

8. *If the initial rhythm is ventricular fibrillation (VF) or pulseless ventricular tachycardia (VT),* warn the examiner to move away from the patient and the trolley, and deliver three shocks in succession: the first and second at 200 J strength; the third at

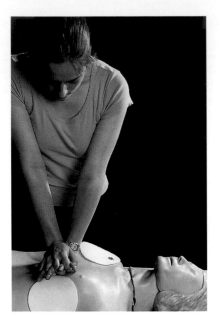

Fig. 5.1.6 Cardiac massage

360 J. Assess the rhythm after each shock to see if you have successfully restored the patient to sinus rhythm.

9. If the dysrhythmia does not revert to sinus rhythm continue CPR at the rate of 15 compressions to 2 breaths. Establish an intravenous (IV) line and secure the airway by endotracheal intubation. Give 100% oxygen through the tube, give 1 mg adrenaline (epinephrine) through the venous access, and continue CPR for 1 minute.

10. If ventricular fibrillation persists, give three direct shocks of 360 J, and check the rhythm after each shock. If the rhythm has not reverted to normal or is non-shockable (i.e. not VT or VF) you might then consider giving 100 mg amiodarone over 10 minutes through the IV line.

11. *If the initial rhythm is asystole,* give 1 mg adrenaline (epinephrine) and a single dose of 3 mg atropine and continue 15 : 2 CPR for 3 minutes. Check if the rhythm has changed to ventricular fibrillation, then follow the protocol for defibrillation as set out in step 8. If still in asystole continue with 3-minute cycles of adrenaline (epinephrine) and CPR. If a slow ventricular rhythm is generated which

does not support the circulation adequately, continue with the CPR until a temporary pacing wire is inserted. Candidates are not expected to proceed to pacing — just explain to the examiner what you would need to do.

12. If the initial rhythm is sinus rhythm (but incapable of producing a cardiac output) in this pulseless, collapsed patient, the diagnosis is *electromechanical dissociation* (now called *pulseless electrical activity*), which has a potentially grave prognosis. You may be asked for its reversible causes: the four 'H's — hypoxia, hypothermia, hyper- or hypokalaemia and other metabolic disturbances, and hypovolaemia — and the four 'T's — tamponade, tension pneumothorax, toxaemia, or a massive pulmonary thromboembolism. (You may also be asked how to correct them.) In practice, this rhythm is treated the same way as asystole, with CPR without defibrillation until a reversible cause is corrected.

Show us, step-by-step, how you would introduce an intravenous cannula into a peripheral vein of this patient.

Gaining intravenous access is an essential procedure that every doctor is expected to be able to do. In many medical schools this procedure is first taught in a clinical skills laboratory on a manikin, before students learn to perform it under the supervision of a House Officer or a Senior House Officer. A manikin, primed with blood, will also be available in the PLAB exam setting, which makes the job easier because the veins do not contract and become invisible due to anxiety, and there is often a visible puncture mark to aim at. However, the procedure is no less daunting on a manikin, as you will be expected to treat the manikin as a real patient, explaining the procedure, and taking all necessary precautions. You must ensure that you have all the required materials and that you explain the procedure to the 'patient' in simple terms.

Explanation to the patient

You should emphasize that the procedure does need to be done, but at the same time reassure the patient. If the patient is anxious he may not want to watch.

> I need to gain access into one of the veins on your forearm or the back of your hand. This means that I have to introduce a needle through the skin into the underlying vein. I am afraid you will feel a prick but these needles are very sharp and they cause as little pain as possible. Try and relax so that your veins do not clam up and hopefully the

procedure can be completed with a single prick. (*Never promise that it will only be a single prick!*) You can look away if you do not wish to see the procedure.

Procedure

Make sure that you have all the materials you require:

- Tourniquet
- Surgical gloves
- Alcohol swabs for skin preparation
- Appropriate size of intravenous cannula (Table 5.2.1)
- 5 ml syringe for saline flush
- Cannula dressing, gauze, bandage, and tape

Remember to take the following *precautions* in this procedure:

- Avoid the veins in the legs, if possible, because these are more prone to thrombosis and infection than those in the arms.
- Never use the arm with an arteriovenous fistula in patients who are on a haemodialysis programme.
- Avoid veins over joints because bending of the joint will interrupt the flow of blood.
- If possible, give the patient the choice of arm. Left-handed patients may wish you to use their right arm for example.
- Take all aseptic precautions during the entire procedure.

Table 5.2.1 Cannula sizes

Size (gauge)	Colour	Use
22	Blue	Small veins IV drugs
20	Pink	Slow fluid administration IV drugs
18	Green	IV fluids Blood transfusion
15	Grey	Rapid IV fluids
14	Brown	Rapid transfusion

1. Wash your hands and wear surgical gloves.
2. Apply the tourniquet above the elbow on the preferred arm and tighten it. Ask the patient to open and close the fist a few times to make the veins visible. Gently tap over the vein to encourage dilatation.
3. Clean the insertion area with an alcohol swab and allow it to dry.
4. Apply traction to the skin with the thumb of the non-dominant hand to fix the vein in place. Hold the cannula with the two wings together and with bevel of the needle pointing upwards.
5. Puncture the skin, holding the cannula at about 15° to the skin, and firmly advance the needle through the subcutaneous tissues into the vein (Fig. 5.2.1). You should get a 'flush-back' of blood into the distal end of the cannula as you enter the vein. Advance it a few more millimetres to get a secure position inside the vein.
6. Hold the cannula steady and advance the plastic cannula over the metal stylet into the vein (Fig. 5.2.2). Remove the tourniquet and the metal stylet (Fig. 5.2.3) and place the cap over the distal end of the cannula (Fig. 5.2.4).

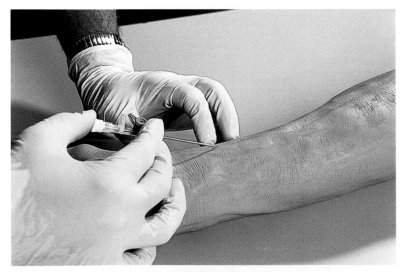

Fig. 5.2.1 Inserting the cannula

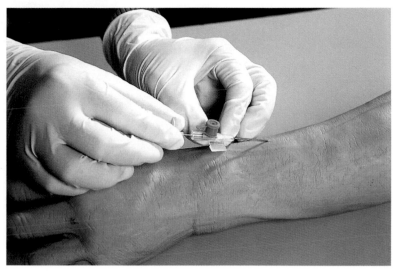

Fig. 5.2.2 Advancing the plastic cannula

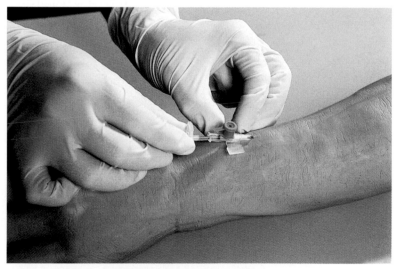

Fig. 5.2.3 Removing the stylet

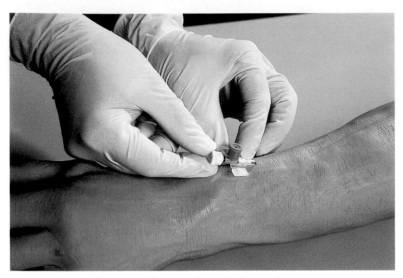

Fig. 5.2.4 The cannula with the cap in place

7. Secure the cannula in place with a dressing and tapes. You may prefer to use a splint and a bandage to guard against accidental removal of the cannula when the patient moves the arm.
8. Instil 5 ml saline in the cannula to flush it, and connect it with a giving set or replace the cap over it until it is required.

Please fill in the laboratory request forms provided and write the appropriate details on the bottles to be sent with them.

After taking blood samples it is essential that you check that both the request forms and the bottles have precise and matching details of the patient from whom the samples have been collected. Most hospitals have pre-printed, self-adhesive addressographs, which you can paste on the request form and the corresponding bottle, but you must still check that the labels belong to the correct patient.

When you collect blood samples from a patient it is sound practice to take all the forms and blood-taking equipment to the patient's bedside. After taking blood all the labelling of the bottles and form-filling can be undertaken at the patient's bedside to eliminate any chance of mislabelling. The request forms for biochemistry, haematology, microbiology, blood bank, and virology are all of different colours and easily distinguishable. These forms should be filled in fully, leaving no questions unanswered. In the exam setting there will be no convenient addressographs and you will need to fill out the request form in full, leaving no blank spaces.

A sample request form

Name	Date of birth	Sex
Address	Ward/Outpatient clinic	Unit number
Date	Time taken	Investigation required
Clinical information	Treatment	

The corresponding bottle must have matching details written clearly on the label:

- Date
- Name
- Address
- Date of birth
- Unit number
- Ward/Outpatient clinic
- Time taken

If a patient is known, or suspected, to have a disease communicable from blood products (e.g. AIDS, hepatitis B/C) this should be marked clearly, both on the request form and the bottle. High-risk bottles should be placed in special high-risk containers and the laboratory should be warned before the samples are sent.

Mrs Jessop is complaining of dizziness on standing. Would you please measure her blood pressure in both sitting and standing positions?

The examiners are looking to see whether you observe all the steps required as you measure the blood pressure.

Explanation to the patient

Whether the subject is a manikin, a volunteer, or a patient, you should explain the procedure as you go along:

> I would like to measure your blood pressure and I need you to rest in this chair for at least 2 minutes before I measure it. (*The patient may, of course, have been sitting for a few minutes before you enter the cubicle.*) I will have to wrap this cuff around your arm and then inflate it. (Make sure that it is of appropriate size for her arm.) It may cause a little tightness around your arm but it should not hurt. Would that be all right? If you have any questions, do please ask me.

Procedure

You will need a stethoscope and a sphygmomanometer. The width of the cuff should be about 40% of the circumference of the arm. The standard size, a 14 cm cuff, should be used for an adult with an average size of arm. Smaller and larger cuffs are available for children and obese subjects respectively. The mercury manometer should be placed at a level corresponding to the heart of the patient to rule out the influence of gravity.

1. Wrap the cuff firmly around the upper arm and secure it so that it does not come undone while you inflate it (Fig. 5.4.1). Feel the corresponding radial pulse as you steadily inflate the

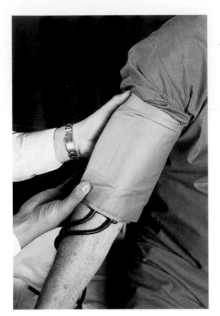

Fig. 5.4.1 A firmly wrapped and secured cuff

cuff (Fig. 5.4.2). As the pressure in the cuff exceeds the *systolic pressure* within the brachial artery the radial pulse will become impalpable. Make a note of this figure and deflate the cuff.

2. Feel the brachial pulse (Fig. 5.4.3) and place the bell of your stethoscope over it in the antecubital fossa. Inflate the cuff to raise the mercury column to the previously noted suprasystolic level. The examiner will be listening simultaneously through the stethoscope, which has four earpieces. As you *gradually* deflate the cuff the passage of blood past the decreasing obstruction creates a series of sounds, the *Korotkoff sounds*, which are audible through the stethoscope. The first loud sound (phase 1) indicates the systolic pressure.

3. As you deflate the cuff the intensity of the Korotkoff sounds will change until they become muffled (phase 4). Note the pressure level at which these sounds disappear (phase 5). This represents the diastolic pressure.

4. Explain to the patient that you will need to repeat this procedure with her standing up. Ask her to hold the sphygmomanometer with her free hand, by her side at the level of her heart. Repeat the three steps above, noting the

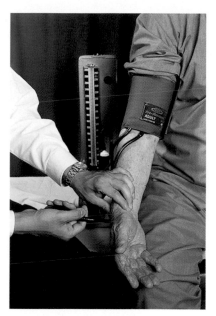

Fig. 5.4.2 Feeling the radial pulse as the cuff is inflated

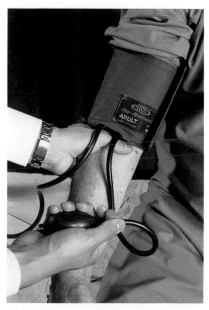

Fig. 5.4.3 Locating the brachial pulse

systolic and diastolic readings with the patient in a standing position. Unless the examiner stops you, check the blood pressure again after 2–3 minutes, as there is a late drop in the standing blood pressure in some patients.

5. Ask the patient to sit down, unwrap the cuff, and replace it neatly in the box. Thank the patient for her cooperation and present your findings to the examiner.

This is Mr Peterson who is complaining of an earache. Please examine his external ear canals and the tympanic membranes with this auriscope.

Explanation to the patient

As always, explain what you are going to do before you begin:

> I have been asked to examine the inside of your ears with this instrument. The procedure should not cause any pain but if there is any discomfort do please let me know. I will gently insert this special lit-up tube in your ear and look through the magnifying glass at the inside of your ears for any signs of infection. Would that be all right?

Procedure

1. Make sure that the auriscope is in good functional order and test the bulb to see that it lights up as you switch it on. Make sure the earpieces are clean and are of an appropriate size for the patient's ear.
2. Look at the external ear for any swellings or scars. Look at the external auditory meatus for any foreign body, discharge, or inflammation.
3. Insert the earpiece and draw the pinna gently upwards and backwards to provide an adequate view of the eardrum (Fig. 5.5.1). If there is no wax or discharge obscuring your view you will see the eardrum, which should look translucent and shiny if it is healthy. You may need to adjust the intensity of the light to get a good view of it. Note if the drum is excessively red, bulging, scarred, or perforated.

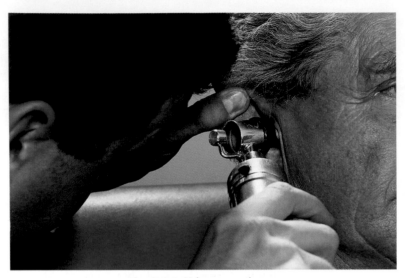

Fig. 5.5.1 Using an auriscope

4. Unless the examiner shows his satisfaction and stops you, you should repeat the procedure on the other side. After completing the procedure switch the light off, remove the earpiece, and set it aside for cleaning.

Please measure the peak expiratory flow rate of this patient.

This is a simple and cheap test for assessing a patient's expiratory performance. Low values are obtained in patients with obstructive airways disease and the test is used to monitor the effect of treatment. A reliable result depends very much on the patient's understanding of what he has to do and on his cooperation. It is therefore important that you explain the procedure and its purpose to him. You may also wish to demonstrate the procedure before asking him to do it.

Explanation to the patient

As the patient's cooperation is so important in this test, make sure that you explain it very clearly:

Using this instrument gives us some idea of how open your airways are and how they are functioning. You have to hold it horizontally like this (*demonstrate this, as in Fig. 5.6.1*) and then take a deep breath in to fill your lungs with air. Hold your breath and tightly purse your lips round this mouthpiece, and then blow into it as much and as forcibly and fast as you can. Take care that all the air goes through the mouthpiece into the instrument and none escapes between your lips and the outer rim of the mouthpiece. You might find it easier if you pinch your nose with the other hand while you are blowing out.

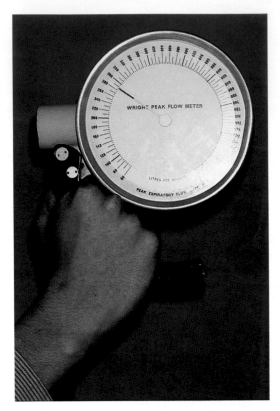

Fig. 5.6.1 Wright's peak expiratory flow meter

Procedure

1. Fix the disposable mouthpiece onto the inlet of the peak flow meter and get the patient to hold it horizontally. Ask him to take a deep breath, purse his lips round the mouthpiece, and blow out hard and fast. See that he is doing it correctly.
2. Get the patient to repeat the procedure twice and select the best of the three readings. Discard the mouthpiece and thank the patient.

Please test this sample of urine with a dipstix.

Routine stix testing of urine is a simple and important investigation for all patients. It is used as a screening test to check the pH and to look for the presence of glucose, ketones, protein, blood, bilirubin, and leucocytes. The reagent test strips on the stix are ready to use straight from the bottle and good results can be obtained by following this simple procedure.

Procedure

1. Make sure that the urine has been freshly collected into a clean, dry container, under sanitary conditions. For stix testing, the urine should be no more than 4 hours old; for a bacteriological examination it should be fresh.
2. Immerse the stix with all its reagent areas in the specimen and remove immediately, wiping any excess droplets against the edge of the container.
3. Hold the strip horizontally and compare the change of colour on each test area against the corresponding area on the colour chart on the bottle label.
4. For a semi-quantitative result, read the reagent areas at the times specified on the bottle label. For a qualitative result, read the reagent areas between 1 and 2 minutes — if positive, repeat the test, reading the reagent chart at the specified time. Record the results on the patient's notes.
5. Remember that colour changes occurring after 2 minutes are invalid.

Imagine that you are going to assist your boss in a surgical operation. You have just scrubbed up in the washroom and you are entering the operating theatre. Show us how you would put on a sterile gown and gloves.

The purpose of this exercise is to see whether you carry out this task observing a strict aseptic technique. Remember that even after a thorough wash your hands are not as sterile as the autoclaved gown and gloves, so your bare hands must not touch anything that is likely to come in contact with the sterile area and instruments during the operation.

Procedure

For this test you will require two sterile towels, a sterile gown, sterile gloves, and an assistant.

Putting on a gown

1. Approach the towels with your forearms semi-flexed at the elbow and the hands held up as if you have just thoroughly scrubbed up.
2. Pick up a towel with one hand and thoroughly dry your hand. Fold it over and sweep it down the arm, drying it to the elbow. Discard it.
3. Take another towel in the other hand and repeat the drying procedure on the other hand and forearm.
4. Pick up the gown and move into an open space with no objects within a radius of 1 m.

5. Open up the gown so that its inside is facing you. Insert both arms into the sleeves and wear the gown over your front, making sure that you keep your hands inside the cuffs of the gown sleeves to allow you to adopt a closed gloving technique.
6. Ask your assistant to tie up the gown from behind.

Putting on the gloves

1. Once your gown is tied up, your assistant will hand you your gloves. With your hands inside the sleeves of the gown, open the glove packet so that the glove fingers are pointing towards you (Fig. 5.8.1). The glove cuffs are turned over to allow you to grasp them and pull them over.
2. Use your right hand (still inside the gown sleeve), grasp the folded cuff of the right glove between your thumb and the forefinger (Fig. 5.8.2), and supinate your hand, still holding the glove. The glove now lies on top of your hand (which is still inside the gown sleeve) with the edge of the rolled-over glove parallel with the gown sleeve (Fig. 5.8.3). You are still

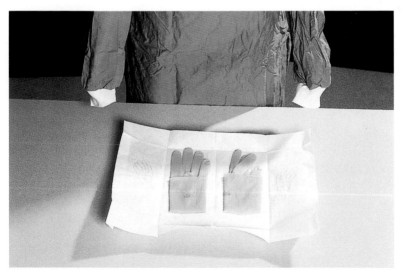

Fig. 5.8.1 Gloves in the starting position

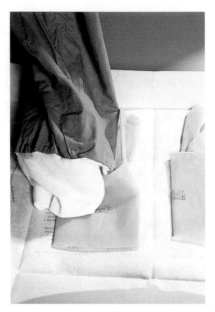

Fig. 5.8.2 Grasping the cuff above the glove thumb

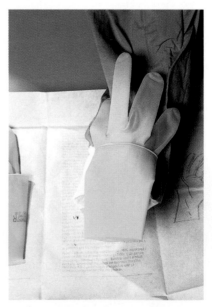

Fig. 5.8.3 The glove turned over

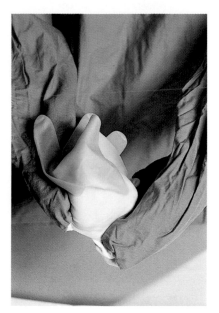

Fig. 5.8.4 Pulling on the right glove

holding on to the glove so that the glove thumb lies below your thumb.

3. With the thumb and the forefinger of your left hand (still in its gown sleeve) pull over the rolled-up cuff of the right glove over the right hand (Fig. 5.8.4). Work your fingers and thumb into the glove, leaving no excess space at the fingertips.

4. Next, with the thumb and forefinger of the left hand (still in the gown sleeve), grasp the rolled-up cuff of the left glove over the glove thumb and supinate your hand so that the glove lies on your hand, as you did for the right hand. With the right hand pull over the rolled cuff over your left hand and work your left hand into the glove (Fig. 5.8.5). Press your finger into the clefts of the fingers of the other hand to ensure that both gloves fit snugly over your hands (Fig. 5.8.6).

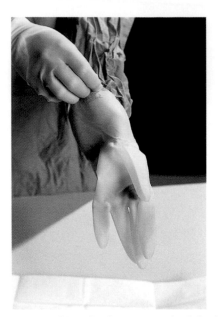

Fig. 5.8.5 Working the fingers into the left glove

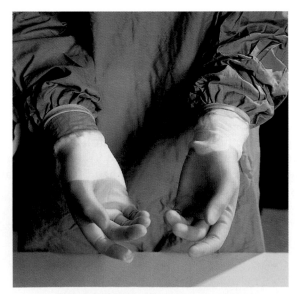

Fig. 5.8.6 Both gloves fitting snugly

Please perform a lumbar puncture on this subject.

The subject is likely to be a manikin but you will be expected to treat it as a real patient, providing it with full information about the procedure and positioning it correctly. A lumbar puncture is frequently required in day-to-day clinical practice and an analysis of cerebrospinal fluid (CSF) is essential for the investigation of a variety of conditions, including meningitis, encephalitis, and subarachnoid haemorrhage. It is a simple and safe procedure and relatively painless (for both patient and doctor) when carried out properly.

Contraindications

- Raised intracranial pressure
- Spinal cord mass lesion
- Local infection at or near lumbar puncture site
- Congenital lesions of the lumbosacral reigon
- Clotting problems

Before proceeding with a lumbar puncture *you must be sure that the patient does not have raised intracranial pressure.* You must confirm this by carrying out fundoscopy, checking that the patient does not have any papilloedema. If there is any possibility of raised intracranial pressure a CT brain scan should be performed before the lumbar puncture.

Explanation to the patient

Once you are satisfied that there is no contraindication, then the key to a successful lumbar puncture is a clear explanation of the procedure to the patient and correct positioning of the patient:

I have been asked to perform a lumbar puncture on you. I expect you have some idea what that entails. Briefly, I will numb a small area on your lower back and insert a needle to get a sample of the fluid that circulates around your brain and spinal cord. You will only feel one prick when I inject the local anaesthetic with this fine needle. You will have to lie on your side with your back at the edge of the bed. The sample of the fluid will give us useful information about the levels of the substances it contains and we will be able to tell whether it contains any bugs. Do you understand what I am going to do, and do you have any questions?

Procedure

Before you start, check that you have all the materials you will require:
- Surgical gloves
- Sterilizing agent
- 5 ml syringe and needles
- 1% lidocaine (lignocaine)
- LP needles
- Manometer
- Three universal bottles
- Sterile dressing

1. Wash your hands and put on gloves. Ask the patient to lie on the bed on his left side with his knees and chin as close to each other as possible. This will maximize the separation of the lumbar vertebral bodies. The presence of an assistant is invaluable — they can encourage the patient to relax and keep his knees drawn up.
2. Identify the third and fourth lumbar spines. The fourth lumbar spine usually lies in line with the corresponding iliac crest. In the exam setting there will be an appliance primed with 'cerebrospinal fluid' in a sitting position, with easily identifiable landmarks (Fig. 5.9.1). Sterilize this area widely up to the iliac crest having made sure first that the patient is not allergic to any of the sterilizing agents or to lidocaine (lignocaine).
3. Empty the contents of an ampoule of 1% lidocaine (lignocaine) into a syringe and then fit it with a small-bore (orange-topped) needle. Inject a small quantity into the dermis between the third and fourth lumbar vertebral spines and raise a bleb. Now fit a pink-topped needle and insert it while injecting more lidocaine (lignocaine).

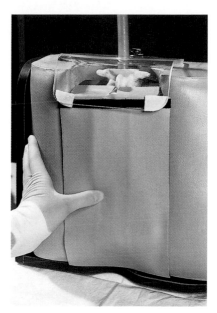

Fig. 5.9.1 Identifying the space between the third and fourth lumbar spines

4. Select an appropriate spinal lumbar puncture needle (assessed according to the patient's size) and pass it through the skin in the midline, pushing it steadily forwards, pointing slightly upwards towards the head of the patient. (Fig. 5.9.2).
5. When you feel the needle has just penetrated the dura mater (there will be increased resistance followed by a sudden 'give'), withdraw the stylet from the needle (Fig. 5.9.3) and allow a few drops of CSF to escape.
6. Connect a manometer to the needle and measure the CSF pressure. The patient's head must be at the same level as the sacrum. (Normal CSF pressure is 60–150 mm H_2O.)
7. Now disconnect the manometer and run its contents into the first sterile container. Collect about 1 ml of CSF in each of the two remaining sterile containers. Check again if you have correctly labelled these containers. An additional sample for measuring the glucose level is also often required (together with a blood glucose sample).

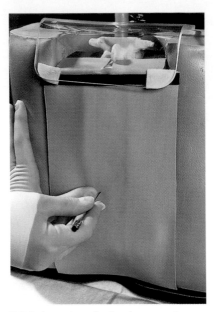

Fig. 5.9.2 Inserting the lumbar puncture needle

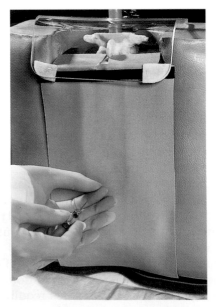

Fig. 5.9.3 Removing the stylet

8. Withdraw the spinal needle and place a sterile dressing on the puncture mark. Ask the patient to lie flat on his back for about 12 hours to reduce the likelihood of headache. Check that all the details of the patient are on the containers and the laboratory request form and send these to the laboratory.

This patient's chest X-ray confirms a left pleural effusion. Please carry out a diagnostic tap.

The patient is most likely to be a manikin and its chest will have been primed with fluid to mimic the real clinical situation, but you will have to behave exactly as you would with a real patient. In a diagnostic tap you are required to obtain fluid to see if it is straw-coloured, haemorrhagic (malignant effusion, pulmonary infarction), or purulent (empyema); send samples for bacteriological and cytological examination; and to aspirate enough fluid to ease the patient's distress if there is a massive effusion.

Explanation to the patient

Explain the procedure to the patient and why he needs it to be done:

> You know that some fluid has accumulated in the left side of your chest. I am going to withdraw some of it, firstly to try and find out the cause, and secondly to take enough of it out to ease your breathing. I will have to insert a needle into your chest to suck out the fluid, but first I will inject a local anaesthetic to make it painless. You will, of course, feel the first prick and a sting when I inject the anaesthetic. If during the procedure you feel any discomfort or pain please do let me know. May I go ahead?

Procedure

Ensure that you have all the materials you need before you start:
- Surgical gloves
- Sterilizing agent

- 5 ml and 50 ml syringes and needles
- 1% lidocaine (lignocaine)
- Scalpel and blade
- Three-way tap and cannula
- Two sterile containers
- Large fluid container
- Sterile dressing

1. Get the patient to sit up on the bed, leaning slightly forwards, with his arms crossed in front, resting on two pillows placed on his lap. Wash your hands and put on gloves.
2. Sterilize the skin over and around the aspiration site, after ensuring that the patient is not allergic to any of the sterilizing agents. You would have percussed over the chest earlier to find the dullest area, where you would insert the aspiration needle. This is usually the seventh intercostal space in the mid-axillary line. Make a little dent with the nail of your index finger in the middle of this space.
3. Draw up 1% lidocaine (lignocaine) in a 5 ml syringe and fit it with an orange-topped needle. Inject a small amount to raise a bleb on the nail mark and insert the needle further, injecting more, thereby anaesthetizing the skin, subcutaneous tissues and pleura.
4. Make a small incision and then insert a brown cannula into the pleural space. Remove the needle and attach to a three-way tap fitted onto a 50 ml syringe. Aspirate about 40 ml and empty the syringe into two sterile containers for laboratory examination. Continue aspiration until you have drained about 1000 ml. You should stop aspiration if the patient becomes uncomfortable. (Shock may ensue if too much fluid is removed too quickly.)
5. Remove the cannula and seal the puncture site with a sterile dressing. Check the details on the request forms and the containers and make sure that these match.
6. Remove the gloves and wash your hands.

Mr Lowe has a right pneumothorax. Please insert a chest drain to decompress it.

This practical procedure is used for the decompression of a pneumothorax, haemothorax, or a pleural effusion. A chest X-ray is essential before proceeding with the insertion of a chest drain. A doctor taking the PLAB exam should be familiar with the procedure, though, to our knowledge, no candidate has been asked to do it in the exam so far. However, it is not beyond the ingenuity of the organizers to produce an appropriate manikin and test you on your competence in this procedure. Alternatively, you may be asked to write down all the steps of the procedure.

Explanation to the patient

Begin by explaining what has happened and what you are about to do:

> Mr Lowe, you know that some air has leaked into the covering membrane of your right lung and that is stopping the lung from expanding fully. As there is a fair amount of air in there I will have to get it out by inserting a drain into your chest about here. (*Point at the second intercostal space in the midclavicular line or the fifth space in the midaxillary line.*) I will inject enough local anaesthetic to make it numb and you will only feel the first prick, and maybe a little discomfort, during the procedure. It sounds worse than it really is. Once the drain is inserted it will be connected through a tube with this bottle, which is fitted with an underwater seal. It will allow the air to bubble away but will not let it back in. The drain will remain in place overnight or even longer until all the air is out of the chest. Is there anything you would like to ask?

Remember to ask him if he is allergic to any of the solutions you are going to use.

Procedure

In the clinical setting you will always find a helpful senior to supervise you, but in the exam you are on your own and you must make sure that you have all the required materials:

- Sterile sheets, gloves, and gown
- Skin preparation solution and swabs
- Local anaesthetic 1% lidocaine (lignocaine), syringe, and needles
- Scalpel, blade, and suture
- Silastic chest drain and underwater seal containing 200 ml sterile water
- One large straight clamp (for drain tubing)
- One curved clamp
- Gauze and tape

Make sure that the patient has adequate intravenous access before starting in case he collapses or has a haemorrhage during the procedure.

1. As you identify the second intercostal space (in line with the sternal angle), make a dent with your nail in the middle of the space in the midclavicular line. This is one of the preferred places for the insertion of a drain but some doctors choose the fifth intercostal space in the midaxillary line. Wash your hands and put on the gown and gloves.
2. The patient should be lying comfortably in bed with the backrest lifted to about 45°. Clean the chest with a sterilizing agent and cover it with drapes, leaving only the intended area of insertion bare. Your nail mark should be visible but make sure that you aim for a spot midway between the second and third ribs.
3. Infiltrate the skin with the local anaesthetic and then the deeper structures, drawing back on the syringe each time you push the needle forward, to make sure that you have not entered a blood vessel. Direct the needle onto the third rib and inject lidocaine (lignocaine) over its superior surface, the periosteum, and the underlying pleura.

4. Make a transverse incision down to the third rib through the anaesthetized area. Using the curved clamp, separate the intercostal structures and complete a blunt dissection with your index finger down to the pleural cavity.
5. *With the trochar removed*, insert the chest tube and direct it with the curved clamp. As you enter a pleural cavity containing air you will notice condensation within the tube from water vapour in the escaping air. (Although trochars are supplied with chest drains they should never be used to introduce the drain as they may cause serious injury.)
6. Connect the tube with the underwater seal and you will notice the initial rush of air as a mass of bubbles.
7. Insert a suture in a circular fashion around the tube to form a purse string, which will be used to close the wound on removal of the drain. Secure the drain with a tape and cover the site with gauze and tape.
8. Remove the drapes, gloves and gown and wash your hands.

Complications

- Haemorrhage
- Damage to intercostal vessels and nerves
- Lung and mediastinal injury
- Allergic reactions

Please carry out a diagnostic peritoneal aspiration on this patient.

A diagnostic tap of ascitic fluid may be required when ascites develops without any obvious cause, such as with portal cirrhosis or an abdominal malignancy. A diagnostic tap is also important if you suspect infection. Aspiration of about 50 ml would be sufficient for a diagnostic procedure, but, occasionally, larger quantities may have to be aspirated to relieve a patient's distress or breathlessness. Repeated aspirations of large quantities, however, result in loss of proteins from the body and the ascites soon reaccumulates unless the underlying condition is remedied.

Explanation to the patient

Start by explaining what you are going to do:

As you know, fluid has accumulated in your tummy. I have to take a sample of it for laboratory examination so that we can find out why this has happened and to see whether it is infected and needs treatment. I will make a small area numb here (*Point to the spot.*) and then introduce a needle and suck out some fluid. Apart from the initial prick and the sting of the local anaesthetic, it should not cause you any pain or distress. Do ask me if you have any questions.

Procedure

Check that you have all the materials you will need:

- Gloves
- Sterilizing agent
- Sterile towels

409

- 5 ml syringe and needles
- 1% lidocaine (lignocaine)
- 50 ml syringe and three-way tap
- Three sterile containers
- Dressing and tape
- 20-gauge cannula

1. Ensure that the urinary bladder has been emptied. Get the patient to lie supine on the bed and make him comfortable, with enough pillows behind his back. Percuss the abdomen, ensuring that one of the flanks is stony dull — this is where you will obtain the fluid from.
2. Wash your hands and wear gloves. Clean the skin with antiseptic and then drape with sterile towels, leaving a small window, about 2 cm square, over the dependent part of the flank of your choice.
3. Infiltrate 1% lidocaine (lignocaine) at the site of the proposed aspiration.
4. Insert a 20-gauge cannula into the skin, remove the needle, and attach a three-way tap connected to a 50 ml syringe.
5. Aspirate 50 ml of fluid and pour it into the three sterile containers (for microscopy and culture, cytology, and biochemistry) on which you have previously written the patient's details. Check the details on the request forms and send these to the laboratory. For symptomatic relief aspirate a maximum of 1500 ml at any one time, as larger volumes may precipitate hypotension and promote further peritoneal fluid accumulation.
6. Remove the cannula, seal the puncture mark with a sterile dressing, and secure it with a tape. Remove the towels and gloves and wash your hands.

Please obtain a bone marrow sample from this patient.

Bone marrow examination is easily performed, carries a negligible risk, and provides valuable information about a variety of diseases. In addition to its usefulness in diagnosis, it provides information on the spread of malignancy, and it may be used to monitor the effects of chemotherapy on haematological malignancies and to evaluate the success of bone marrow transplantation.

In the UK, haematologists usually carry out this procedure after a clinical assessment of the patient and examination of the blood count and peripheral blood film. The major *contraindication* to bone marrow aspiration is haemorrhage or local infection at the site of puncture. Thrombocytopenia alone is not a contraindication, but a full blood count and clotting screen should be carried out before commencing the procedure.

A doctor in the second year after graduation would be expected to be familiar with the procedure, and you may be asked to perform it on a manikin in the exam. The examiners will be looking not only at your technique, but also whether you know what equipment you would need and how you would explain the procedure to the patient.

Explanation to the patient

This must sound a formidable procedure and no one would anticipate it without some understandable anxiety. You should take this into account and reassure the patient that you will use a generous amount of local anaesthetic to minimize the pain caused by the entry of the needle into the marrow space. You should concede that there will be some discomfort caused by the pushing and prodding and by the actual aspiration of the

marrow (which can be distressing). This should be done while
you explain the various steps that will be required to obtain the
marrow aspirate. You will need the assistance of a nursing
colleague who will help you with the procedure and provide
support and reassurance to the patient.

Procedure

You will require the following equipment:

- Clean trolley
- Sterile gloves
- Skin preparation (iodine or chlorhexidene)
- Sterile dressing towels, swabs and gauze
- 1% plain lidocaine (lignocaine)
- 5 ml and 10 ml syringes
- 19-gauge and 21-gauge needles
- Bone marrow aspirate needles (with a guard, either Salah or Klima)
- Clean microscope slides and spreader
- Media and containers for specialized tests and cultures

The posterior iliac crest is used in both adults and children.
The body of the sternum may be used if the subject is obese and
the iliac crest is inaccessible, or if the patient is unable to lie on
her side. Aspiration may also be taken from the anterior iliac
crest or from the lumbar vertebrae. For the posterior iliac crest
approach the patient is placed in the right lateral position with
the back flexed.

1. Wash your hands and wear sterile gloves. Identify the bony
   landmarks and clean the skin. Surround the area of the ilium
   lateral to the posterior superior iliac crest with sterile towels.
2. Infiltrate the skin, subcutaneous tissues, and particularly the
   periosteum, with 1% lidocaine (lignocaine). Assemble the
   aspiration needle with stylet and guard. The guard may be
   removed for iliac crest procedures but is essential for sternal
   puncture — it should be screwed 1–2 cm from the tip of the
   needle and adjusted so that only a further 5 mm advancement
   is possible once the periosteum is reached.
3. Hold the needle at a right angle to the skin and advance it
   until the periosteum is reached. Maintaining the needle at a
   right angle, advance it towards the bone, using a clockwise and

counter-clockwise action to push it through the outer cortex of the bone. As the marrow cavity is reached you will feel a sensation of decreased resistance.

4. Remove the stylet and attach a 10 ml syringe. Apply sharp suction and aspirate up to 0.5 ml of marrow — any larger a volume would lead to contamination of the sample with peripheral blood. Marrow for ancillary tests should be taken into a separate syringe once the slides have been prepared. If no marrow is aspirated on the first attempt, rotate the needle or replace the stylet and cautiously advance or retract the needle. If marrow is still unobtainable a different site should be attempted.

5. Smear the aspirate on slides quickly before it clots. It is important to obtain good smears as badly prepared specimens are difficult to interpret. Place single drops of aspirated marrow onto slides, tilting them to allow the blood to drain away. Make the films using a smooth glass spreader. Satisfactory slides must include blood as well as marrow particles. At least eight slides should be prepared for staining: Romanowsky and iron stains should be carried out routinely and further cyto- and immunochemical tests may also be required. All slides should be fixed and any unfixed slides should not be stored. Gloves should be worn at all times during the preparation of slides. Only aspirate marrow for additional tests after the slides have been prepared and quickly place it into an appropriate medium (usually anticoagulant, unless for microbiology).

6. Remove the towels and gloves and wash your hands.

Complications

- *Haemorrhage.* Usually seen in patients with severe coagulation disorders. This may be limited by ensuring that any coagulation disorders are fully corrected before the procedure.
- *Bony perforation.* This occurs more commonly when performing sternal aspiration. Failure to use the guard may lead to complete penetration of the bone, resulting in potentially life-threatening complications. Perforation is more likely in patients with osteoporosis or with malignant infiltration of the marrow.
- *Infection at the site of aspiration.* This is rare as long as an aseptic technique is rigorously followed.

Please obtain an arterial blood sample from this patient for blood gas analysis.

Blood gas analysis is an important investigation and provides invaluable information about the level of oxygen and the carbon dioxide tension in the blood, and about the overall metabolic status of the body. Reliable results are crucially important in the clinical assessment of patients whose cardiorespiratory status or metabolic equilibrium is compromised. Errors in blood gas analysis may arise from incorrect sampling techniques, or from careless storage and transport to the laboratory. Some basic principles must be understood and strictly followed in order to minimize these.

Precautions

1. *Analysis.* The sample obtained should either be analyzed immediately, or the syringe, having been sealed with a plastic cap, should be stored in ice before and during its transfer to the laboratory. Ideally, the laboratory should be warned about its arrival and an assistant should be ready to take the sample as soon as it is obtained. If the sample is left waiting in an ambient environment, unimpeded white cell metabolism consumes oxygen and increases the carbon dioxide level.
2. *Anticoagulation of the sample.* The sample must be adequately anticoagulated to prevent clot formation within the analyzer. However, excessive dilution with heparin will falsely reduce the pH. As a rule of thumb, approximately 0.1 ml of heparin should adequately anticoagulate a 2 ml sample.
3. *Air bubbles.* Invariably, a few air bubbles enter the syringe but they should be expelled as soon as possible, as they may lead to falsely high oxygen levels in the sample.
4. *Inspired oxygen levels.* The sample should be taken when the patient is breathing room air, but if he is on oxygen then the

inspired oxygen concentration should be taken into consideration when interpreting the results.

Explanation to the patient

Although this is a simple procedure, often requiring only a single needle prick, its purpose and method should be explained to the patient. He may experience more discomfort or pain than he would in venepuncture as arterial punctures can be more intrusive and painful. He should be offered a local anaesthetic, though this is seldom necessary. You will also need his cooperation in keeping perfectly still while you are attempting to enter the artery.

Procedure

1. You have the choice of the radial, brachial or femoral arteries (but avoid the latter in young children for fear of spasm or thrombosis). For a radial or brachial arterial stab, ask the patient to keep his arm straight and supinated on the bed or a side table. Clean the area with a swab where you feel the pulse.

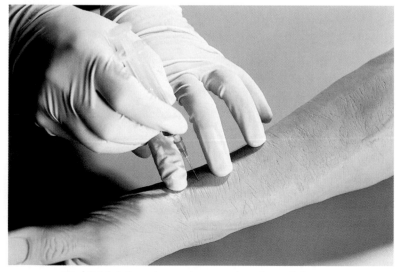

Fig. 5.14.1 Locating and puncturing the radial artery

415

2. Feel the radial pulse with your left index and middle fingers while steadying the patient's hand with the remaining fingers and the thumb. Just distal to the midpoint of your finger, where you feel the maximum pulsation, insert a vertically held 23-gauge needle on a 2 ml syringe (Fig. 5.14.1). As you feel you have pierced the artery, withdraw about 1.5 ml of blood. Withdraw the needle and get the patient to apply firm pressure on the site of puncture while you expel the air bubbles from the syringe.
3. Seal the syringe with a plastic cap, place it on ice, and get it transferred to the laboratory as soon as possible. Examine the puncture site and press on it for a few minutes. Apply a dressing to the puncture site.

Introduce a central venous catheter by cannulating the right subclavian vein in this patient.

Subclavian vein cannulation is an important practical procedure which is sometimes a life-saving measure, for example for temporary pacing in complete heart block. It is used for central venous and pulmonary capillary wedge pressure measurements in heart failure, and for parenteral nutrition in severe malnutrition or where oral feeding is not possible. Every clinician should master the technique of subclavian cannulation because it provides quick central venous access in any state of vascular collapse. It is a simple technique and, performed with care, need not cause any complications.

Explanation to the patient

Explain the procedure to the patient and encourage him to ask any questions he might have:

We need access to your central venous system (*or the right side of the heart*) and we do this by inserting a needle here, below your collarbone. Apart from a prick and some stinging it should not cause you any pain. However, during the procedure you have to lie flat without any pillows. I hope that is not going to cause any discomfort — it will only be for a short time. Is there anything you would like to ask?

Procedure

Start by checking the equipment you need:

- Sterile gloves
- Swabs and sterilizing agent

417

- 5 ml syringe and needles
- 1% lidocaine (lignocaine)
- Scalpel and blade
- Syringe and 20-gauge needle
- Catheter and guide wire
- Suture
- Gauze and tape

1. Wash your hands and wear gloves. Get the patient to lie supine, with the head tilted down by about 5°, to avoid air embolism.
2. Clean the skin and infiltrate the skin below the midpoint of the right clavicle with 1% lidocaine (lignocaine). Make a 3 mm nick on the skin with the scalpel to ease the entry of the needle (Fig. 5.15.1).
3. Introduce a 20-gauge needle on a 10 ml syringe beneath the clavicle and first rib and aim at the suprasternal notch (Fig. 5.15.2). *It is of critical importance that you keep the needle as close to the undersurface of the clavicle as possible, and advance it towards the suprasternal notch in order to enter the subclavian vein.* If you have difficulty in aiming the needle correctly, get an assistant to place the tip of his index finger in the suprasternal notch.
4. If you are in the vein, blood will flow freely into the syringe as you withdraw the plunger. Remove the syringe and introduce the guide wire through the needle into the subclavian vein (Fig. 5.15.3).

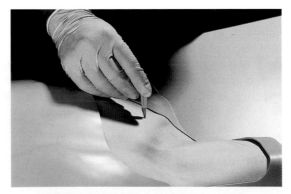

Fig. 5.15.1 Incision at the entry point

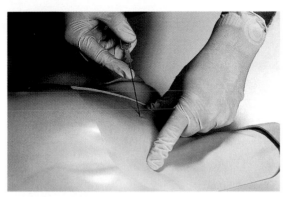

Fig. 5.15.2 Directing the needle towards the manubrium

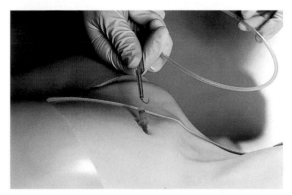

Fig. 5.15.3 Introducing the guide wire

5. Remove the needle, leaving the guide wire in the vein, and then pass the catheter over the guide wire into the vein (Fig. 5.15.4). Advance the catheter so that its tip lies approximately in the distal part of the superior vena cava.
6. Remove the guide wire (Fig. 5.15.5) and secure the catheter firmly with a suture. Place gauze over the catheter and secure it with tape.
7. Request a chest X-ray to confirm the position of the catheter.

Complications

■ *Subclavian arterial puncture.* If you suspect that you have entered the artery and blood pulses into the syringe, remove the needle quickly. The arterial puncture will close spontaneously and there may be no further problem.

419

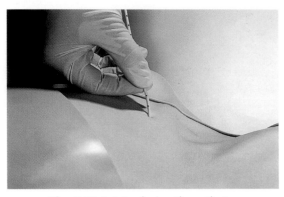

Fig. 5.15.4 Introducing the catheter

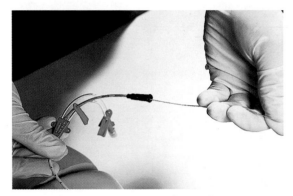

Fig. 5.15.5 Removing the guide wire

Occasionally, this results in a haemorrhage and the entry wound should be pressed on firmly for a few minutes.

- *Pneumothorax.* This is rare but may be large enough to require aspiration.
- *Air embolism.* This can be avoided if the patient's head is kept lower than his trunk, and the index finger is placed on the hilt of the needle when the syringe is removed.
- *Thrombosis.* A minor degree of thrombosis may occur if the procedure takes longer than a few minutes, but major thrombotic episodes causing pulmonary thrombosis are rare.
- *Catheter-related sepsis.* This can be avoided by using a strict aseptic technique, but may occur as a late complication and should be borne in mind if the patient develops septicaemia.

Insert a catheter into the internal jugular vein of this patient.

Some internists prefer internal jugular vein cannulation to a subclavian approach and sometimes, for one reason or another, the latter procedure may be unsuccessful. The average postgraduate doctor is expected to be proficient in both techniques. The materials required are the same as for the subclavian vein cannulation, and the procedure should be explained to the patient in the same way.

Procedure

1. Place the patient supine on a bed with his head tilted down so that the neck veins become distended.

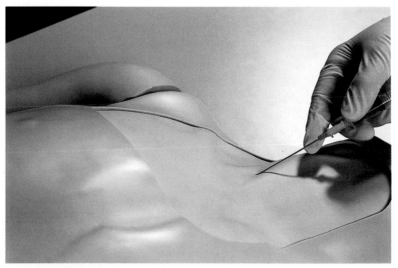

Fig. 5.16.1 Aiming for the internal jugular vein

2. Clean the skin over the neck and make sure that the procedure remains sterile throughout.
3. Inject 1% lidocaine (lignocaine) intradermally at the apex of the triangle formed by the two heads of the sternomastoid muscle and the clavicle. Make a 3 mm incision with a scalpel.
4. Insert a cannula on a syringe through the incision and direct it laterally, downwards, and backwards (Fig. 5.16.1) until you puncture the internal jugular vein, just beneath the skin and deep to the lateral head of the sternomastoid. Draw the plunger to check that blood flows freely into the syringe.
5. Introduce a guide wire through the cannula into the vein and then remove the cannula.
6. Introduce a venous catheter over the guide wire into the vein and remove the wire (see Fig. 5.15.5; p. 420). Secure the catheter with a suture and place gauze and tape over it.
7. Request a chest X-ray to confirm that the catheter tip is in the superior vena cava and to check for any pneumothorax.

Outline and demonstrate the various routes by which a therapeutic substance can be injected into a patient's body.

The purpose of this instruction seems to be to find out not only whether a candidate is proficient in giving an injection, but also, more importantly, whether he can educate a patient in the art of self-injection. Injection is defined as the act of giving medication by syringe and needle. There are nine major routes through which this objective is achieved:

1. Subcutaneous
2. Intramuscular
3. Intravenous
4. Intradermal
5. Intralesional
6. Intra-arterial
7. Intra-articular
8. Intracardiac
9. Intrathecal

Intrathecal routes are employed when the prescribed drug is unable to cross the blood–brain barrier. Site selection is predetermined for intra-articular, intrathecal, intracardiac, intra-arterial and intralesional injections. These routes of administration are used when specific therapeutic effects are required and should be carried out by an experienced individual, as they have serious and potentially life-threatening complications. The choice of remaining sites will depend on the desired therapeutic effect and the patient's safety and comfort.

The main sites used for *subcutaneous injections* are the lateral aspects of the upper arms and thighs, the abdomen in the umbilical region, the back, and the lower loins. Slow absorption is a priority so ideal sites are those that are poorly supplied with sensory nerves and blood vessels. Site rotation reduces the possibility of irritation as a result of frequent use. This technique is used by diabetic patients to provide them with a regular supply of insulin and by patients who require long-term low molecular weight heparin.

Five major sites are used for *intramuscular injections*:

1. *Mid-deltoid.* Used for injection of narcotics, sedatives, tetanus toxoid, vaccines and vitamin B_{12}. It is easily accessible and is the best site for small-volume, rapid-onset injections.
2. *Gluteus medius.* This has the lowest drug absorption rate and is used for deep intramuscular injections. May be complicated by sciatic nerve or superior gluteal artery injury.
3. *Gluteus minimus.* Best used for injections of large volumes and for injections in elderly and emaciated patients as it is away from any major neurovascular structures.
4. *Rectus femoris.* Used for antiemetics, sedatives, and narcotics. It is the preferred site in children and for self-administration.
5. *Vastus lateralis.* Used for deep intramuscular injections. It is a large muscle, free from any major vascular structures, can be used for large-volume injections, and accommodates repeated injections.

Explanation to the patient

This is an important part of the exercise. Simple though the task seems, its purpose and execution should be explained fully to the patient. Reassure the patient that the needles used for injections are very sharp and cause only a minor prick at the point of entry. Warn the patient that there will be some discomfort when the material is injected.

Procedure

In order to perform a subcutaneous or intramuscular injection you will require the following equipment:

- Clean tray
- Any protective clothing that may be required
- Patient's prescription chart to check dose and route
- Skin cleansing solution or alcohol swabs
- Sterile syringe containing the drug to be injected
- Sterile needles of varying length
- Sterile cotton wool

Subcutaneous injection

Expose and prepare the site with cleansing solution. Choose the correct size of needle and, with the skin gripped firmly, insert the needle into the skin at an angle of 45°. Release the gripped skin. Pull back the plunger and, if no blood is aspirated, inject the drug slowly. If blood does appear, withdraw the needle and begin again. On completion, withdraw the needle and apply firm pressure before safely disposing of your equipment.

Intramuscular injection

Explain the procedure and help the patient into the appropriate position. Expose and clean the chosen site. Choose an appropriate needle, based on the patient's weight. Stretch the skin around the site and plunge the needle at a 90° angle quickly into the skin, leaving a third of the shaft exposed. Pull back the plunger and, if no blood is aspirated, slowly inject the drug. If blood does appear, begin again. On completion, withdraw the needle rapidly and apply pressure before safely disposing of your equipment.

Intravenous injection

Intravenous drug therapy is used for patients where an immediate therapeutic effect is desired. Intravenous therapy requires a more accurate dose calculation and is free from the potential pain and irritation caused by subcutaneous and intramuscular injections.

There are three main methods of intravenous drug administration:

1. Continuous infusion
2. Intermittent infusion
3. Bolus administration

The mode of intravenous drug administration depends on the nature and volume of the drug to be administered. The method that you will be most frequently directly involved in is the bolus method of drug administration.

Bolus intravenous injection

This procedure may be carried out through the injection site of an intravenous administration set, via an adaptor or injectible plug into a cannula, or via an extension set, multiple adaptor, or stopcock (one-, two-, or three-way). Check that you have the necessary equipment:

- Clean tray containing the drug to be administered
- Patient's prescription chart
- Sterile needle and syringes
- Saline- or heparin flush ready for injection

Explain the procedure to the patient. Wash your hands and check if there is an infusion in progress. Make sure that the drug is appropriately prepared. Prepare the saline or heparin flush for injection. Place all the equipment on a clean tray. Before administering the drug, inspect the cannula site and check its patency with the flush. If there is an infusion in progress, switch it off. Inject the drug smoothly and slowly, either directly into the cannula or into an attached plug or adpator. On completion, reapply the flush and ask the patient if she is experiencing any discomfort. If more than one drug is to be administered, flush the cannula with saline between each drug. On completing the drug administration ensure that the patient is comfortable, restart any infusion that was in progress, and complete the patient's prescription chart.

Please pass a nasogastric tube in this patient.

Passing a nasogastric tube is a simple and sometimes life-saving procedure which every doctor must be able to do. The procedure is fairly straightforward on a manikin, but in real life it may be difficult if there is any narrowing of the oesophagus or if the patient is unable to cooperate. As the task is relatively easily accomplished on a manikin, the examiners will watch your technique closely, to judge whether you would be successful on a real patient who might have some difficulty in swallowing. They will note whether you check for the common pitfalls, such as passing a tube deceptively easily, only to find it has curled up inside the mouth.

Explanation to the patient

Passing a tube through someone's nose into the pharynx can be an unpleasant experience and may generate bouts of coughing, frustrating both the doctor and the patient. It is important to explain the necessity for such a procedure and to reassure the patient that if he makes an effort to swallow the tube as you advance it, you will be able to pass it quickly and without much distress. Ask him to be ready with a glass of water and a straw.

Procedure

You will need the following equipment:

- Nasogastric tube — large-bore for aspiration, and small-bore for feeding
- Non-sterile gloves and apron
- Kidney dish
- Water-soluble lubricant

- Glass of water and a straw
- Pen torch
- 20 ml syringe
- Universal indicator paper
- Draining bag

Once you have everything ready and have explained the procedure to the patient, start by checking that you have an appropriate tube.

1. You can decide whether you have a tube of the right length by using it to measure the distance from the nose to the tragus of the ear, and from there down to about 5 cm below the costal margin in the midaxillary line. A nasogastric tube of about 50 cm is usually adequate for an adult.
2. Put on the gloves and apron, and keep the kidney dish nearby in case the patient vomits. Get him to sit upright with his neck slightly flexed. Lubricate 10 cm of the advancing end of the tube and insert it into the patient's nostril.
3. Aiming at the patient's occiput, advance the tube slowly. It may induce a gag reflex as it enters the oropharynx. Ask the patient to swallow a sip of water as you advance it further.
4. Ask the patient to open his mouth and shine a pen torch in to see if the tube is in the pharynx or only lying curled up in the mouth. Withdraw and reintroduce the tube if it has become curled up in the mouth or higher up in the nasopharynx.
5. Ask the patient to swallow another sip of water, and advance the tube gently down the oesophagus. If at any stage the tube does not progress further, you should stop and get him to swallow another sip of water to aid peristalsis.
6. Advance the tube further until it has reached the predetermined distance.
7. Connect the tube to a syringe and aspirate. If the tube is in the stomach the aspirate will contain stomach contents. Test the pH of a drop of the aspirate on universal indicator paper — a pH of 4 or less indicates the presence of gastric contents.
8. If the patient is taking any anti-acid formulation (e.g. proton pump inhibitors, H_2-receptor antagonists, antacids), the pH of the gastric contents will not be acidic and you may be in doubt about whether the tube is in the stomach. Using the

syringe, inject some air into the tube while your assistant auscultates over the stomach for gurgling sounds.

9. If you are still in doubt obtain an X-ray to confirm the placement of the nasogastric tube in the stomach.
10. Tape the tube to the nose. Attach the drainage bag to the nasal end of the tube.

Please obtain an aspirate through a fine needle from this swelling.

Fine needle aspiration (FNA) provides material for cytological analysis, and so diagnostic evaluation, of cystic and solid masses. It is particularly important in the evaluation of thyroid masses. It is a safe and relatively simple procedure that can be conducted relatively quickly on the ward or in the outpatient clinic.

Explanation to the patient

Explain the procedure and its purpose, using simple terms:

The only way we will know the nature of this swelling is if I can aspirate a bit of it by using a fine needle. I will use a local anaesthetic first, to numb the skin where I insert the needle. You will only feel the initial prick and a sting from the anaesthetic. Through this fine needle I will suck up a little material from inside the swelling which we will send to the laboratory for a detailed microscopic examination.

Procedure

Check that the following equipment is on your tray or trolley:

- Sterile gloves
- Skin cleansing preparation (iodine or chlorhexidene)
- 1% lidocaine (lignocaine)
- Selection of needles — 21-, 23-, and 25-gauge
- 10 ml syringe
- Glass slides for preparation
- Sterile cotton wool
- Dressing

1. Clean and prepare the skin over the lesion to be aspirated. Inject 1% lidocaine (lignocaine) at the site of aspiration.
2. Attach an appropriate size of needle to the 10 ml syringe and insert it at an angle of 90° into the swelling. Gently aspirate, ensuring that you do not obtain blood as this will make cytological analysis difficult. If you do obtain blood, withdraw the needle, apply pressure, and start again.
3. Place the aspirated material on a clean glass slide, which should then be placed in a slide holder. Repeat this procedure two to three times to ensure adequate sampling of the lesion.
4. On completion, withdraw the needle, apply pressure for a minute, and then apply an adhesive plastic dressing over the needle mark. Label the prepared slides clearly and send them to the cytology laboratory with the appropriate request forms.

Please carry out a urethral catheterization on this male patient.

In the exam setting you will be required to do this on a manikin, but the necessary explanation to the patient, the equipment you need, and the strict aseptic technique should all be as they would be for a real patient.

Explanation to the patient

You should explain the need, purpose, and details of the procedure to the patient in simple and easily understandable terms. For example, he may have been unable to pass urine and may be in some distress and in need of relief, or you may have to test his kidney function by measuring precisely how much urine he is making. You should reassure him that the procedure may appear unpleasant or may cause some discomfort but that you will be gentle and will try not to hurt him.

Procedure

Check that you have all the materials you require:

- Clean trolley — make sure it has been swabbed with alcohol and allowed to dry
- Assistant
- Catheterization pack
  - Gauze swabs
  - Kidney dish
  - Drapes (sterile towels)
  - Forceps
  - Cotton balls
  - Plastic dish

- Sterile gloves
- Sterile cleaning solution
- Tube of lidocaine (lignocaine) jelly
- Foley catheter — a size 14 is usually adequate. For problematic or long term catheterization, a silastic catheter should be used
- 10 ml syringe and 10 ml sterile water

1. Draw the curtains round the patient's bed and ask him to lie in a supine position.
2. Wash your hands thoroughly. With the trolley by the side of the patient, have all the equipment ready on it. Get your assistant to open the catheterization pack without touching any of the contents. Put on the gloves aseptically, without touching the outside of them with your fingers.
3. Drape the patient's pelvis with sterile towels, leaving only the penis exposed. Get your assistant to pour the cleaning solution in a plastic dish.
4. With your non-dominant hand, gently retract the foreskin and clean the urethral orifice and the glans with the cleaning solution using the same hand, leaving the other hand sterile for catheter insertion.
5. Warn the patient that you are going to squeeze a local anaesthetic inside his urethra and that, although it will sting a little at the beginning, it will make the passage of the catheter virtually painless. Squeeze the contents of the tube of lidocaine (lignocaine) jelly (approximately 20 ml) into the urethra and gently massage the ventral surface of the penis to aid the passage of the jelly further down the urethra.
6. Open the catheter wrapping at the insertion end of the catheter and place the other end in the kidney dish. Insert the catheter into the urethral meatus and advance it gently into the urethra using the sterile forceps (Fig. 5.20.1).
7. As the catheter tip enters the urinary bladder, urine will flow back into the kidney dish. Advance the catheter another 2–3 cm to ensure that the balloon lies inside the bladder.
8. Through the side tube that is connected to the balloon, slowly inject sterile water to inflate the balloon that will anchor the catheter inside the bladder (Fig. 5.20.2). Watch the patient's face carefully in case the balloon is still inside the urethra and causes pain, in which case you should deflate it by withdrawing the water before advancing it further.

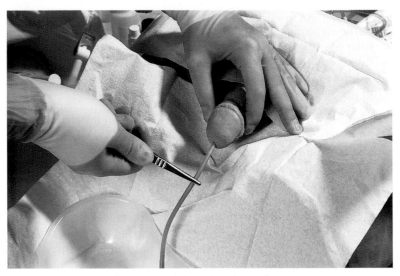

Fig. 5.20.1 Advancing the catheter

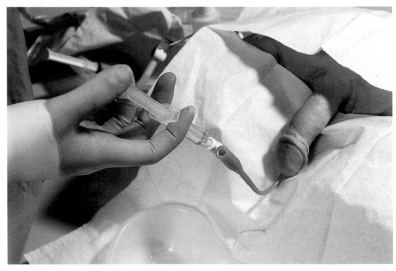

Fig. 5.20.2 Inflating the anchoring balloon

9. Once the balloon has been inflated, pull back on the catheter until you feel the resistance of the balloon against the neck of the bladder. Attach the catheter to the collection bag and record the volume of urine obtained.
10. Protract the prepuce back over the glans to avoid the risk of paraphimosis.
11. Remove the drapes and restore the patient to his normal position in bed.
12. Remove the gloves and wash your hands.

Please carry out a urethral catheterization on this female patient.

The equipment and explanation would be the same as for male urethral catheterization, but extra sensitivity is required with regard to patient privacy and delicacy. Ideally, a female doctor or nurse performs urethral catheterization in a female, but all male doctors should be familiar with the procedure as they may be called upon to do it in an emergency. *Male doctors must be accompanied by a female chaperone*, who can also provide some help in explaining the procedure to the patient and act as assistant in the procedure. Catheterization of females is easier than catherterization in males, as they have a shorter urethra and no prostate to impede the passage of the catheter.

Procedure

1. The position of the patient is the same as for obtaining a cervical smear (see p. 438). Make sure that the patient is relaxed, in a supine position, with her knees bent and abducted and her feet together.
2. Dip a swab in the cleaning solution and clean the labia majorum on one side from above downwards. Discard this swab and use a fresh one for the other side. Similarly, use two swabs for cleaning the labia minora from above downwards. Clean the urethral orifice with the fifth swab.
3. Drape the patient with sterile towels, leaving only the labia minora exposed. Insert the lidocaine (lignocaine) gel as for male catheterization.
4. Get your assistant to unwrap the outer covering of the catheter and deposit it in the sterile kidney dish.

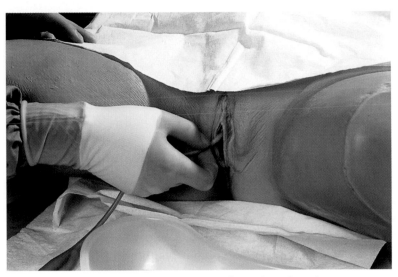

Fig. 5.21.1 Checking the catheter is anchored

5. Hold the catheter pack, expose the catheter and insert it in the urethra without touching it. While still holding the pack, advance the catheter gently till it enters the urinary bladder. The rest of the procedure is the same as that for male catheterization. Check that the catheter is securely anchored with the sterile hand after you have inflated the balloon (Fig. 5.21.1).

Would you please take a cervical smear from this patient?

The patient in this case is always a manikin but you should be fully cognizant of such a situation in a clinical setting, and should take care to mention that you would require the presence of a *chaperone* and that you would explain the procedure to the patient.

Explanation to the patient

Find out if the patient has had a similar procedure in the past and explain it in simple terms. Explain that it is a 3-yearly check-up, for which a scraping is taken from the neck of the womb, via the vagina. Ask for her permission and reassure her that there will be a female nurse present during the entire procedure.

Procedure

Check that you have all the equipment you require:

- Surgical gloves
- Good illumination
- Bivalve vaginal speculum (different sizes)
- Spatula (Aylesbury or Ayre)
- Slide with ground-glass end
- Fixative
- Slide mailer
- Lead pencil
- Request form
- Ballpoint pen

1. Put the patient's name and number on the ground-glass end of the slide, using a lead pencil (other markers are washed off

by processing fluid). Check the details and write a pathology request form. Make sure that the wooden spatula you use is free from splinters, splits, and other defects. Have the fixative ready. Wash your hands and put on surgical gloves.

2. In the exam there will be a manikin, reasonably well placed for the task. Position the light. Choose the correct size of speculum and warm it with a little tap water. Do not use a lubricant or antiseptic. Warn the patient before you insert the speculum into the vagina, and secure it so that it remains in place and you have an adequate view (Fig. 5.22.1). Observe the patient's face for any pain or discomfort.

3. Insert the spatula into the cervical os using the bi-lobed end (Fig. 5.22.2). Use the spade end if the cervix is patulous or scarred. Do not clean the cervix or wipe away any attached mucus until the smear has been taken. Firmly rotate the spatula through one and a half turns, ensuring that the scrape spans the squamocolumnar junction at all points (Fig. 5.22.3). Remove the spatula and speculum, cover the patient, and thank her for her cooperation.

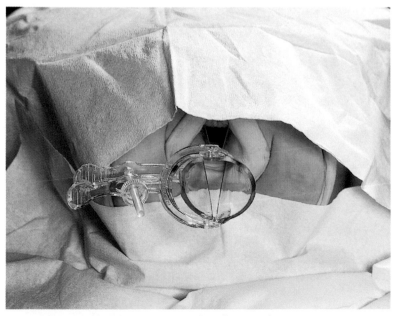

Fig. 5.22.1 Inserting the speculum

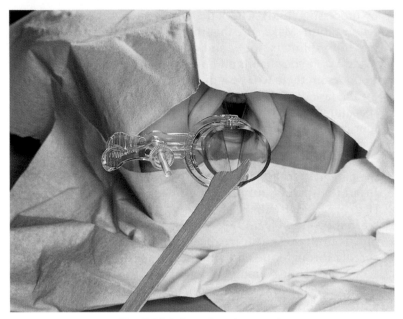

Fig. 5.22.2 Inserting the spatula

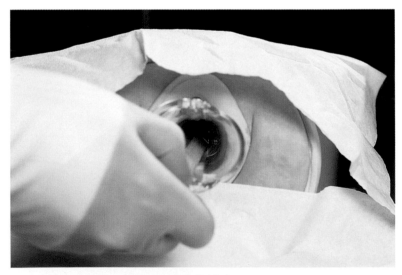

Fig. 5.22.3 Taking a smear

4. Spread the material thinly on the glass slide, using gentle, longitudinal strokes. The aim is to spread a single cell layer over as much of the slide as possible, without damaging the cells.
5. Place the slide on a horizontal surface and immediately apply a generous amount of fixative. Pour off any excess after a few minutes and allow to dry for 10 to 20 minutes.
6. Put the slide into a container for the laboratory.
7. Remove your gloves and wash your hands.

This is Mrs White (a manikin). She is 34 weeks pregnant. I would like you to perform an obstetric examination on her.

The examiner has given you a specific task and the spotlight will be on your obstetric abdominal palpation skills. First, however, you should introduce yourself to the patient and exchange pleasantries. Enquire about the general state of her health and about fetal movements.

Obstetric abdominal examination

Begin with a general inspection, assessing uterine enlargement, symmetry, scars, and the linea nigra. The height of the uterine fundus may be assessed either using a tape measure (symphysis—fundus height) (Fig. 5.23.1), or by feeling the distance of the fundus from the xiphisternum.

Palpation

The purpose of palpation is to determine the position of the fetal head; to assess the fetal size and whether it is compatible with the dates; and to assess the amount of liquor amnii. Ask the patient if any area hurts and reassure her that you will be careful. Use the palm of the hands, not the fingertips, for palpation.

Fundal assessment
Facing the patient, place your left hand along the right lateral aspect, and your right hand along the left lateral aspect of the fundus of the uterus (Fig. 5.23.2). This method will allow you to feel the fundus and its contents and will give you a reasonable idea of the quantity of the amniotic fluid present.

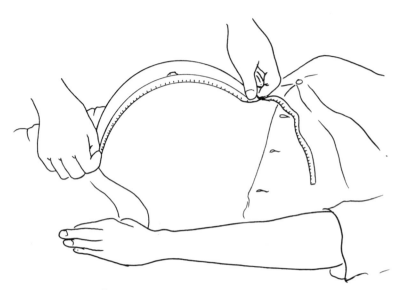

Fig. 5.23.1 Measuring the fundal height

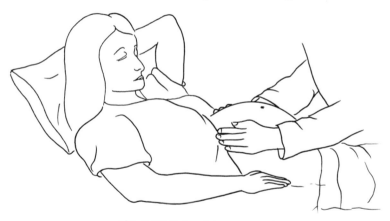

Fig. 5.23.2 Fundal assessment

Lateral assessment

Facing the patient's legs, place your left hand along the left side of the lower abdomen, and the right hand along the right lateral aspect of the uterus (Fig. 5.23.3). Palpate with the whole length of your palms while you watch the patient's face for any discomfort. Explain to the examiner that systematic 'dipping'

443

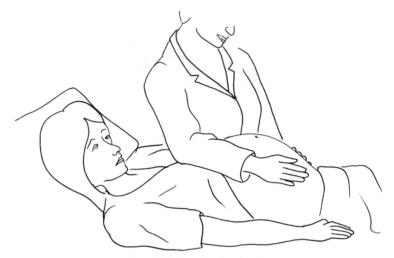

Fig. 5.23.3 Lateral palpation

palpation (to displace the amniotic fluid) from the right side towards the midline will reveal either the firm resistance of the fetal back, or fetal limbs.

Pelvic/lower-segment assessment
While still facing the patient's legs, slide your two hands gently down to feel the uterus at the pelvic brim. If the *lie* is longitudinal, the head (or breech) will be palpable over the pelvic inlet. If the lie is oblique (i.e. the long axis of the fetus at an angle of 45° to the long axis of the uterus) the presenting part will be palpable in the iliac fossa.

After completing the abdominal palpation, auscultate the fetal heart. Use a sonic aid or a special fetal stethoscope and listen over the fetal back for the heart sounds (Fig. 5.23.4). Examine the legs for oedema and varicose veins, and test the urine for protein and glucose.

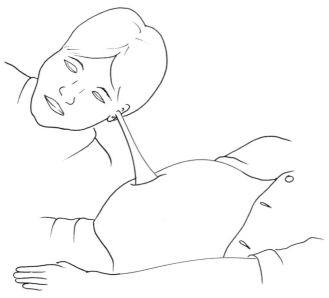

Fig. 5.23.4 Listening for fetal heart sounds

Please suture this open wound.

At this station you will find a manikin arm or leg on which a
neat incision has been made, separating the two flaps that you
are to suture together. You may even see the perforation marks
of the previous candidate's suturing. In real life, the main
objective is to repair the wound aseptically and neatly so that it
heals by first intention, leaving a linear scar that, with the
passage of time, could be mistaken for a skin crease or a
wrinkle. When you suture the two flaps together you should
ensure, therefore, that they are neatly apposed and not
overriding each other.

Explanation to the patient

In clinical practice, explaining this procedure is reasonably easy
because the patient comes with a laceration and knows that it
will need to be sutured. Nonetheless, it is important to explain
the objective and the procedure to the patient and to warn him
that it will cause some pain.

Procedure

Sutures

Sutures may be either *non-absorbable* sutures, which are used for
skin closure and have to be physically removed (e.g. nylon,
polypropylene, and silk) or *absorbable* sutures, used for suturing
wounds in mucous membranes and deeper tissues (e.g. catgut,
vicryl, and dexon). It is important to select the appropriate size
of thread. The coarser the thread, the lower the number (0, 1, 2);
the finer the thread, the higher the number (5/0, 6/0). Different
sites require sutures of different sizes:

- Skin on the arms and legs — 3/0 and 4/0
- Face and the back of the hand — 5/0 and 6/0
- Skin over major joints in adults — 3/0
- Most other sites — 4/0

Before you start, check your equipment tray:

- Sterile gloves
- Needle holder
- Sutures
- Non-toothed forceps
- Scissors

1. Wash your hands and wear sterile gloves.
2. Put sterile drapes round the incision (or wound) to be sutured.
3. Unless the examiner asks you to put in continuous sutures, you should employ the usual method of instrument-tied interrupted sutures. Hold the needle holder in your dominant hand and grasp the curved needle about one-third of its length away from the end connected to the thread. The needle should be held perpendicular to the needle holder.
4. Starting about 0.5 cm away from one end of the wound, insert the needle through the skin at right angles to the incision, to enter the opposing edges (Fig. 5.24.1). You may find it easier

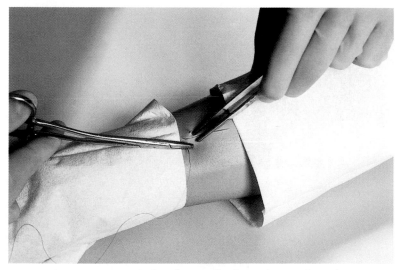

Fig. 5.24.1 Introducing the needle through opposing edges

if you apply counter-pressure with the forceps on the opposite side of the wound.

5. Glide the needle through both flaps of the incision and exit at a point equidistant from the entry site. With the forceps, pull the needle and thread through without snagging (Fig. 5.24.2).

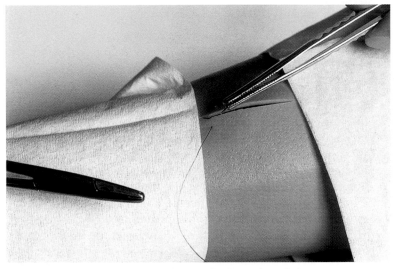

Fig. 5.24.2 **Pulling the needle through with forceps**

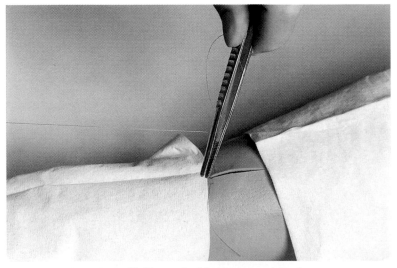

Fig. 5.24.3 **Making a double loop round the forceps**

6. The two suture ends must now be tied with the formation of a knot — wrap the opposite strand twice clockwise round the needle holder or the forceps (Fig. 5.24.3), and then pull the end of the opposing strand through the loop (Fig. 5.24.4), making a square knot (Fig. 5.24.5).

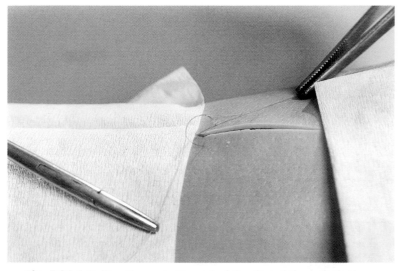

Fig. 5.24.4 Pulling the opposite end of the thread through the loop

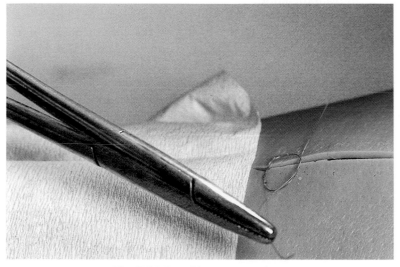

Fig. 5.24.5 Making a square knot

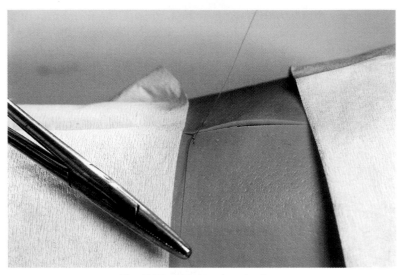

Fig. 5.24.6 Tightening the knot

7. Now pull the two strands together to tighten the knot
   (Fig. 5.24.6). In order to secure this knot and make sure that it
   does not slip, repeat the procedure, this time making the
   double loop anticlockwise. Tighten the second knot over the
   first, so making a square knot, and cut both strands about
   1 cm from the knot.
8. The distance between the interrupted sutures should be
   roughly twice the thickness of the edges being sutured. About
   0.5 cm away from, and parallel to, the first suture, insert the
   needle again and repeat steps 4 to 7. Continue to suture up
   the wound, making sure that all the knots lie on the same side
   and that the cut ends are of the same length.
9. At the end wipe the sutured line clean with sterile gauze and
   apply a sterile dressing.

Please complete Part 1 of this cremation form.

The cremation form is a legal document required to confirm the deceased's identity and the cause of death. As no further examination can be undertaken on the deceased after cremation has taken place, this document must show that there was no foul play and that the deceased died of a natural cause as stated on the death certificate. You should be mindful of these requirements when you complete Part 1 of the document. Completion of the form is a straightforward exercise as long as you are the person who was involved in the care of the deceased during his or her final illness, and you either filled in the death certificate yourself or are in agreement with the cause of death as stated by someone else. Even though, in the exam setting, there will not be a deceased person available for identification, you must satisfy the examiners about your knowledge of the following points:

1. If you did not certify the patient's death you will need to visit the mortuary to identify the deceased about whom you are going to complete Part 1 of the cremation form.
2. You need to be sure that the patient has no radioactive implants or a permanent pacemaker fitted.
3. The cause of death written on the cremation form must be the same as that on the death certificate. If you did not certify the death you will need to see the case notes and satisfy yourself about the cause of death. You may need to discuss it with the doctor who issued the death certificate.
4. You should have been the patient's medical attendant during their final illness, and you will need to state the length of that period of care in the appropriate section of the form.
5. It is usually members of the nursing staff working on the patient's ward who cared for the patient in their terminal illness, and who were present at the time of death. This answer

would be sufficient to complete the relevant sections of the form.

6. As you will receive a fee for completing the first part of the cremation form, it is important that you keep a record of the forms you complete, as you will be liable to pay tax on this income.

Outline the essential requirements for writing a concise and informative discharge letter.

The discharge letter is an important part of a patient's management following an admission to hospital and needs to be written clearly and concisely. It provides information for both the general practitioner and for other physicians who may be involved in the patient's further management, either immediately after discharge or subsequently. Consequently, a discharge letter needs to outline the patient's diagnosis, investigations, management, and drugs prescribed on discharge, as well as plans for future follow-up. You will need all the patient's notes and results of investigations in front of you as you prepare to write the letter.

The letter needs to be clear and concise, maximizing the amount of useful information it contains. It should be written according to the following sub-headings:

1. Patient details
2. Admission and discharge dates
3. Primary and subsidiary diagnoses
4. Inpatient investigation, management, and progress
5. Discharge medication (The diagnosis and the discharge medication and dosage are the most important factors and must be written clearly, legibly and in full.)
6. Follow-up plans (This should include the next proposed clinic appointment and any further investigations planned as well as any referrals made to specialist colleagues.)

Telephone calls

Introduction

The telephone is an important instrument of communication, not only between a doctor and other health care workers, but also between doctors and the public and the media. A doctor may have to refer a patient; discuss a problem with a specialist; inform a senior colleague about an urgent situation; respond to an enquiry from a relative; or talk to inquisitive reporters. As the telephone is so important in planning patient management, there is at least one station in most exam centres where candidates' telephone communication skills are tested.

You may be asked to conduct a telephone conversation with a patient, an anxious relative, a nurse, your consultant, or a consultant of another speciality. You may be given a script and you should be able to answer the questions asked by the other party from the information you are given. In your answers you will have to address the issues raised and you will have to make a clinical decision based on the information you have been given. Your task may be to ask an anxious mother to bring her child to hospital; it may be a request to your consultant to come and see a patient; or you might have to ask your house officer to arrange an X-ray. Even though there may not be a functional telephone at the station, or the person supposed to be at the other end of the telephone may be sitting right in front of you, you must conduct the conversation as you would in a real-life situation. You should practise with a colleague so that you learn to remain calm, maintain a moderate tempo, and get into the habit of tackling the most pertinent points efficiently.

In this section we have described six scenarios to give you some idea of what sort of problems are presented and what may be expected of you. As in the history and counselling sections, there is a wide range of cases that could be presented, but we hope that these examples illustrate what to expect and how to approach this type of station.

From a mother to a doctor in Casualty

You are the SHO in the Casualty Unit and an anxious mother of a 3-year-old child calls you on the telephone. She says that her child is hot, restless, and crying, and that she has found a rash on his left leg. Please take a relevant history from her and advise her what she should do.

In this situation you should calm the caller and attempt to get enough relevant details to enable you to make a decision on what you should advise her to do. This is not the time to get a very detailed history, as a lengthy conversation is only going to increase her anxiety and make her feel that nothing is being done. The story suggests that this child probably has meningococcal infection and will require urgent treatment, but if you tell her to bring in the child without asking her any questions she may panic. In the exam station there will be an actress with a telephone, pretending to be ringing from home.

Mother: Hello, hello, is that the Accident and Emergency Department?

Doctor: Yes, you are through to Casualty. How can I help you?

Mother: Hello! Are you a doctor? I am in dreadful trouble. I don't know what to do.

Doctor: Yes, this is Dr Rana speaking. Please be calm and tell me exactly what the trouble is. Try to speak slowly and clearly.

Mother: Oh, doctor, I don't know what to do. My little boy is ill. I don't know what is wrong with him. Can you help me?

Doctor: Please don't worry. I'll do all I can to help you. First of all, please tell me your name and telephone number in case this line gets cut off. Yes, thanks, I've got it Mrs Craig. Now, tell me, how long has your little boy been ill?

Mother: Only since this morning, doctor. Last night he was champion but this morning he feels hot and he's gone off his food. I don't know what's wrong with him. He is inconsolable, crying all the time.

Doctor: Mrs Craig, how old is he?

Mother: Tom is 3 years old. He's never had any trouble, apart from an odd cold in the winter but he is much hotter and more irritable than he's ever been before.

Doctor: Does he have any other symptoms, such as vomiting or a headache?

Mother: No, he hasn't been sick, but he's got a rash on the outside of his left leg.

Doctor: Could you describe it for me, please? Are there only a few spots on the side of the leg, or are there other spots on the back of the leg or anywhere else?

Mother: No, just a few spots on the outside of the leg. I looked all round him and there are no more spots.

Doctor: What colour are they? They are dark red, are they? All right. Are they raised? Can you feel them (*palpable purpura*)?

Mother: No, doctor.

Mother: Do they fade when you press on them?

Mother: Yes, doctor, they do fade when I press over them.

Doctor: (satisfied that there is a rash) Mrs Craig, it looks as if little Tom has an infection. There is no need to worry — it is treatable. We will need to see him here, however, and give him treatment straightaway. Once you are here I will explain it in more detail. Please give me your address and I will arrange an ambulance to fetch you both here. I will make sure that the ambulance gets there within the next 20 minutes. Right, I've got your address. Just wait there, but keep him cool — you could rinse a couple of towels under the tap and sponge his arms and legs down to lower his temperature a little. Make sure the water is not too cold. Did you get that? OK, I'll see you soon. Bye.

From the SHO to her consultant

You are the SHO on a surgical ward and you and the nursing staff have been stabilizing a patient who collapsed at about 11.30 p.m. You contact your consultant, give him the details of the patient and his present condition, and ask him to come and see the patient.

In this scenario the examiner will play the role of the consultant, who will be on the other side of the screen and you will speak to him while holding a telephone (although he can hear you anyway). This time you will have a script. The examiner may ask you a question for which you have no scripted answer but it should be possible to deduce the information you need from the given details.

The patient, Mr Beecham, is a 50-year-old man who was admitted that morning with absolute constipation. A high colonic obstruction was suspected and a hemicolectomy was performed. The operation was uneventful and he was stable until about 11.30 p.m. when he suddenly collapsed. You suspect a haemorrhage and think that the anastomosis needs to be explored.

Doctor: Hello, Mr Hudson. Good evening. This is Dr Mathur, your SHO. I am very sorry to call you at midnight. I hope I haven't got you out of bed.

Consultant: No, I was up anyway. Don't worry. What is the matter?

Doctor: I need to talk to you about a patient, Mr Beecham, who was admitted this morning and had a hemicolectomy performed by Mr Catherick. Our firm is on call this evening and I was called half an hour ago when he collapsed with a blood pressure of 80/50 mm Hg. His pulse was 120 beats per minute, temperature was 37.4 °C, and he had a respiratory rate of 30 per minute. On examination, he looked pale and anxious. His abdomen was rigid and there was a leakage of blood at the operation site. I have given him fluids and antibiotics, and have put up a unit of blood. I have sent blood samples for arterial blood gases, U&Es, full blood count, and LFTs. I have requested six units of blood to be crossmatched. His ECG is normal and he is being monitored.

Consultant: I don't know Mr Beecham. Could you tell me something more about him?

Doctor: He is 50 years old. He was admitted this morning with absolute constipation. A lump was felt in the left hypochondrium and they suspected that he had a tumour in the descending colon. This was confirmed on a CT scan of the abdomen. A hemicolectomy was done and his progress was uneventful until he collapsed at 11.30 p.m. I suspect that he is bleeding from the operation site.

Consultant: What would you like me to do?

Doctor: I am sorry to bother you, but the Specialist Registrar is doing an appendicectomy and I think this man needs to go back to theatre pretty soon. I would be grateful if you would come and have a look. I have already informed Sister in theatre, and the anaesthetist and I have discussed it with Mrs Beecham and obtained her consent in case we need to operate again. I have started the blood transfusion and more is on its way.

Consultant: OK, I will be there in half an hour. Chase the lab for the results of his gases, FBC, and urea and electrolytes. Continue the transfusion and keep him stable.

Doctor: Will do. Thank you very much.

Consultant: All right. Bye.

Doctor: Bye. See you soon.

From a House Officer to the SHO

You are the SHO on call and you have just stabilized a patient who was admitted with an exacerbation of his chronic obstructive pulmonary disease. You and your house officer carried out the necessary investigations (full blood count, urea and electrolytes, arterial blood gases, chest X-ray, etc.) and started the patient on antibiotics and continuous oxygen. He was comfortable when you left him, but no sooner have you reached your room than your house officer called you to say that the patient has suddenly become very breathless.

The house officer, played by the examiner, has a script from which he will answer your questions. You have to choose the questions that should explore your differential diagnoses and then make a decision about the management of this patient.

HO: Hello, Tim. I am sorry to ring you so soon, but Mr Slater has taken a turn for the worse. He has suddenly become breathless for no apparent reason — at any rate, I can't find one.

SHO: No problem, Bob. What about his pulse and BP?

HO: His pulse rate is 100 per minute. It was 90 per minute when you left him. His BP is stable at 150/90 mm Hg. He looks well otherwise, apart from some understandable anxiety.

SHO: What about any other symptoms? Does he have any wheeze, cough, haemoptysis, or chest pain?

HO: No, none of those. He's still bringing up some mucopurulent sputum but it is not streaked with blood. I thought of a pulmonary embolism but there is no evidence of that. His cardiac state is stable and his calves are soft and non-tender, and not swollen. I suppose it is still possible and I was thinking of starting him on heparin, anyway.

SHO: Yes, we may have to do that but we must try to find a cause of his breathlessness if we can. How about an arrhythmia or a myocardial infarction?

HO: The monitor did not show any change in his rhythm. His ECG does not show any change from his last tracing which was 6 months ago.

SHO: You examined him and you can't find any new signs?

HO: No. He is just breathless, in spite of the oxygen and reassurance.

SHO: Bob, remind me, what were his FVC and his PEFR when they were last tested?

HO: His FVC 6 months ago was 1.6 litres and his PEFR today was 160 litres/minute.

SHO: I think Mr Slater has popped one of his bullae and has a small pneumothorax. It will be too small to be detectable clinically, but large enough to compromise his already meagre respiratory reserve. You arrange an urgent chest X-ray, and I am on my way.

The ward sister to the SHO

You are the SHO on a medical firm and you have just put up a blood transfusion on a 60-year-old woman, Mrs Perkins, who was admitted with melaena and whose haemoglobin level was 8 g/dl. As soon as you reach your room, the ward sister rings you to tell you that Mrs Perkins has rigors and is pyrexial. She wants to know whether this is the result of some kind of mismatch of the blood and if she should stop the transfusion.

You have to address the concerns expressed by the ward sister (who will be played by an actress) and make a decision about the appropriate next step.

Sister: Hello, Dr Klinsky. Sorry to bother you, but I don't like the look of Mrs Perkins. Just about 10 minutes after we started the transfusion she developed pyrexia, with a temperature of 38°C and she is shivering.

SHO: Did you check the details on the blood pack? Do they match with Mrs Perkins' particulars?

Sister: Yes, we did. Everything checks — the name, age and the unit number.

SHO: Does she have any other symptoms? Any itching, or a rash?

Sister: No, just the rigors and a temperature and both of these started soon after we began the transfusion. As you know, she was apyrexial on admission. Do you think it is a mismatch, or could she be allergic to something in the blood? I have reduced the rate of transfusion — but should I stop it altogether?

SHO: No, Sister. Please don't stop it. As her symptoms started so soon after the transfusion, I think it is a pyrogen reaction. Please give her 300 mg of aspirin and I will come and see her.

Sister: Aspirin? Are you sure? Don't you think she has some infection?

SHO: No, I don't think so, but I will take some blood samples for culture when I get there. The aspirin will reduce her temperature and settle her rigors. See you soon, Sister. Thank you.

From a caller who claims to be a relative of a patient, to the SHO

In this scenario you are the SHO and you get an outside call from a man who says he is Mr Albert Shelling, the brother of Mr Brian Shelling. The latter is a patient who is under your care with had a stroke, and Mr Albert Shelling is enquiring about his condition.

An actor will play the role of 'Mr Albert Shelling' and he will be speaking from the other side of the screen. He will ask his questions from a script and you have to choose appropriate answers and make a decision about his request.

Caller: Hello, doctor, good evening to you. Am I right in thinking that you are the doctor looking after my brother, Mr Brian Shelling? I am Mr Albert Shelling.

SHO: Yes, I am Dr Al Rawi and Mr Brian Shelling is a patient of mine.

Caller: How is Brian doing? Could you tell me something about his present condition?

SHO: I'm afraid I am not at liberty to give any details about a patient to an unknown caller on the telephone. I think I am right in saying that you have not been to the hospital to see Mr Shelling, and I don't know you. I am not even sure that you are who you say you are. Could you tell me something that I can verify from Mr Shelling's notes — perhaps his address, or telephone number?

Caller: That is very proper of you, if I may say so. But I have a problem. You see, I have not seen my brother for 15 years, since I moved to the Isle of Skye. We have not been in touch and I don't know his current address or his telephone number. A mutual friend of ours rang me only today to say that Brian had had a stroke and that he had been admitted to hospital. It took me some time to find the telephone number of the hospital and the name of the doctor I should speak to. So, please could you just tell me how he is doing? I am very anxious about him. You appreciate, he *is* my brother even though we haven't met for many years.

SHO: Under the circumstances I suppose there is no harm in telling you that Mr Shelling had a left-sided stroke 3 days ago, but he is making good progress. We are transferring him to the Stroke Unit tomorrow where he will get more intensive physiotherapy. His rapid progress so far suggests that he should make a complete recovery.

Caller: That is very good news, thank you. I am sure he is in good hands. You have been very kind and I can't thank you enough. Please can I make one other request?

SHO: What would that be?

Caller: Could you give me his son's address, please, so that I can write to him?

SHO: I'm afraid I can't bend the rules that far. I can't give you any of his personal details, even if I was certain that you are his brother.

Caller: I thought I had made my position quite clear. I have lost touch with my brother and surely you can understand that I would like to write to my nephew. He could do with some sympathetic support at the moment.

SHO: I'm afraid it is one of the rules of this hospital that we must not divulge any personal details of a patient or of a member of staff to anyone on the phone.

Caller: Rules be damned!

SHO: Mr Shelling, I did not make the rules. I am only trying to follow them. I can't give you his son's address or his telephone number.

Caller: That is really irritating, and you call yourself a compassionate doctor! I have a right to know my nephew's address. How on earth do you think I can get in touch with him?

SHO: By visiting your sick brother in hospital and meeting your nephew. Is that not possible?

Caller: No, that's just it. My business commitments mean that I can't get away from here at the moment. But I would like to drop a line to my nephew. How do you suppose I can do that?

SHO: I can't give you the address of young Mr Shelling but I can solve your problem.

Caller: How?

SHO: You give me your address and telephone number, and I will pass these on to your nephew and ask him to ring you. I will tell him that you are keen to get in touch with him. You can then ask him anything you wish. Surely that would solve your problem?

Caller: If that's all you can do, don't bother. I will find some other way. Thanks for nothing!

From the SHO to the on-call radiologist

You are the SHO in Casualty and you have just completed your assessment of a 75-year-old woman, Mrs Appleton, who was admitted in a confused state from a residential home. The carer accompanying her has told you that Mrs Appleton is forgetful and confused; that she has difficulty in walking, so much so that she has fallen a few times; and that her son, out of kindness, smuggles in alcohol for her which she drinks when she goes to bed. On examination, you found that she has poor orientation and recall, that she is unsteady on her feet, and that she has an upper motor neurone weakness in her right hand. You have to persuade the on-call radiologist to perform an urgent CT scan of her brain.

The examiner will play the role of the reluctant radiologist. His questions are not all answered on your script but there is enough information on it for you to make your case.

SHO: Hello, Dr Bligh, Good evening. I am sorry to ring you so late in the evening. I am Dr Sharma, the SHO on call in the Casualty. I need an urgent brain scan on a patient here.

Dr Bligh: Tell me about the patient.

SHO: This is a 75-year-old woman brought in from a residential home. She drinks alcohol and has dementia. On examination I found her to have an unsteady gait and weakness in the right hand.

Dr Bligh: Why do you want to put this old dear through a CT scan at this time of night? She has probably had a stroke and if a scan *must* be done, then it can surely wait till tomorrow morning.

SHO: I'm afraid not. I think she may have a haematoma and may need urgent treatment.

Dr Bligh: Well then, get a neurosurgeon to see her and if he wants a brain scan he can ask for it.

SHO: I am now in a catch-22 situation — you would like a neurosurgeon to see her before you do a CT scan, but a neurosurgeon would want a scan before he sees her. I was just trying to save time. Besides, I could make a convincing case for the neurosurgeon to see her.

Dr Bligh: What makes you think she has a haematoma? What kind of a haematoma would it be anyway?

SHO: Her confusion and unsteadiness are aggravated by her alcoholism. Apparently, her son surreptitiously brings in the supplies because he thinks it is the only pleasure she has. However, her weakness in the right arm only started a few weeks ago, after she had a fall. I think this lady has a chronic subdural haematoma.

Dr Bligh: OK. I am on my way. You've convinced me. Your lady will have a CT scan of the brain after all!

SHO: Thank you.

Index